THERAPEUTIC MASSAGE & BODYWORK

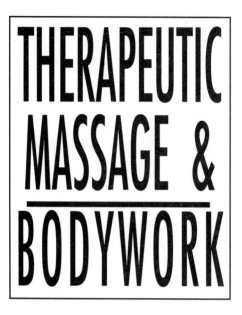

THERAPEUTIC MASSAGE & BODYWORK

Second Edition

750

Questions & Answers

Jane S. Garofano, PhD, NCTMB

National Certification of Therapeutic Massage and Bodywork
Owner/Director
JSG School of Massage Therapy

Associate Professor of Biological Sciences
Bergen Community College
Paramus, New Jersey

APPLETON & LANGE
Stamford, Connecticut

Copyright © 1999, l997 by Appleton & Lange

All rights reserved. This book, or any parts thereof, may not be used or reproduced in any manner without written permission. For information, address Appleton & Lange, Four Stamford Plaza, PO Box 120041, Stamford, Connecticut 06912-0041.

97 98 99 00 01 / 10 9 8 7 6 5 4 3 2 1

Prentice Hall International (UK) Limited, *London*
Prentice Hall of Australia Pty. Limited, *Sydney*
Prentice Hall Canada. Inc., *Toronto*
Prentice Hall Hispanoamericana, S.A., *Mexico*
Prentice Hall of India Private Limited, *New Delhi*
Prentice Hall of Japan, Inc., *Tokyo*
Simon & Schuster Asia Pte. Ltd., *Singapore*
Editora Prentice Hall do Brasil Ltda., *Rio de Janeiro*
Prentice Hall, *Upper Saddle River, New Jersey*

ISBN 0-8385-0337-3

Acquisitions Editor: Jessica Hirshon
Production Service: Inkwell Publishing Services
Production Editor: Meredith Phillips
Designer: Mary Skudlarek

PRINTED IN THE UNITED STATES OF AMERICA

This book is dedicated to my family: Neil, Julie and Paul, Mom and Dad, and to those who helped me decide on pursuing my interest in therapeutic massage and bodywork; and achieving my goal to open the JSG School of Massage Therapy for Healthcare Professionals

Contents

Preface

Appleton & Lange's Quick Review: Therapeutic Massage & Bodywork, Second Edition has been designed and revised according to the guidelines of the National Certification Exam for Therapeutic Massage and Bodywork (NCTMB), which is administered throughout the United States, Canada, and Puerto Rico. This review book enables the applicant to review relevant material while becoming familiar with the types of questions given on the exam. Each question has one answer and a brief explanation with references provided at the end of each practice test. Although the questions are scrambled, they are coded as to content:

M = Massage and Bodywork   AP = Anatomy and Physiology
P = Pathology   B/E = Business/Ethics

This feature helps identify content areas that require further study. The book is divided into four Practice Test sections of 150 *content coded* questions with answers, explanations, and references. A Comprehensive simulated examination is also provided at the end of the book.

All areas of therapeutic massage and bodywork are covered in 600 questions that closely correlate in percentage to the new National Certification Examination content areas outlined in the NCTMB Candidate Handbook. The new content is divided into Human Anatomy, Physiology, and Kinesiology (27%), Massage/Bodywork Theory, Assessment, and Practice (41%), Clinical Pathology and Recognition of Various Conditions (20%), and Business Practice/Ethics (12%). Within these content areas, more topics relevant to non-Western bodywork and holistic touch therapy modalities as well as ethics and clinical pathology are included and outlined below.

I. Human Anatomy, Physiology, and Kinesiology (27%)
    A. Western
        1. Major systems: location and function

- Integumentary system
- Skeletal system
- Muscular system
- Nervous system
- Endocrine system
- Cardiovascular system
- Lymphatic and immune system
- Respiratory system
- Digestive system
- Urinary system
- Reproductive system
- Craniosacral system

2. Biomechanics and kinesiology
- Efficient and safe movement patterns
- Proprioception
- Basic principles of biomechanics and kinesiology

3. Basic medical terminology

B. Non-Western

1. Traditional Chinese medicine
- Primary meridians and organ physiology
- Extraordinary meridians—conception and governing vessels
- Five element theory

2. Other energetic systems

II. Clinical Pathology and Recognition of Various Conditions (20 percent)

A. History and client intake process

1. Emotional states and stress leading to disease
2. History of abuse and trauma related to disease and recovery
3. Impact of client medical history on disease and recovery
4. Effects of life stages on basic health and well-being

B. Disease and injury-related conditions

1. Signs and symptoms of disease of the major systems of the body: indications and contraindications
2. Physiological changes and healing mechanisms

III. Massage Therapy and Bodywork Theory, Assessment, and Practice (41 percent)

A. Assessment

1. Effects of gravity
2. Integration of structure and function

      3. Use of palpation for assessment of craniosacral pulses, energy blockages, and bony landmarks

      4. Somatic holding patterns in clients

      5. Using visual cues in assessing clients

      6. Conventional Western medical approaches to client's illness

      7. Structural compensatory patterns

      8. Interview techniques

  B. Application

      1. Sites to avoid on client's body

      2. Proper client draping and positional support

      3. Physiological and emotional effects of touch on client

      4. Effective and appropriate responses to client's emotional needs

      5. Universal precautions

      6. Use of appropriate verbal and nonverbal communication skills

      7. Physiological changes brought about by touch therapy

      8. Practitioner's self-awareness during a session

      9. Using strategies to plan single and multiple client sessions

      10. Use of manual contact and manipulation to affect soft tissue, joints, and the energy system

      11. Use of joint mobilization techniques

      12. Use of terms related to quality of movement

      13. Using and teaching basic principles of posture and kinesthetic awareness

      14. Hydrotherapy

      15. CPR and first aid

IV. Professional Standards, Ethics, and Business Practices (12 percent)

  A. NCTMB Code of Ethics

  B. Confidentiality of client information

  C. Effective interprofessional communication

  D. Use of proper income-reporting procedures

  E. Basic business and accounting practices

  F. Session record-keeping practices

  G. Scope of practice: legal and ethical parameters

    The last section of the review book contains a Comprehensive Simulated Exam of 150 questions selected from the previous bank of questions and answers. Since the actual exam is uncoded, so is this. There are

150 multiple choice questions also available on the disk packaged with this book. The exam is given by an electronic testing system; therefore, the disk is included to practice the test on a computer in the three-hour period provided at the testing center. The answer key follows; the explanations are found in the previous sections.

The reference list includes all the books recommended by the NCTMB, as well as a few additional resources that include recent and relevant material that should be referred to during review.

Study Strategy

Before attempting the questions in the review book, a thorough knowledge of anatomy and physiology is essential, particularly of the bones, muscles, blood vessels, and nerves. All methods of therapeutic massage and bodywork, including individual strokes and meridians, as well as prominent people that are associated with the methods, are important to know. It is also necessary to have an understanding of the ethical and business philosophies. Review draping techniques and personal hygiene. Be familiar with the ailments, injuries, and diseases that can benefit from therapeutic massage and how to treat them along with any first aid needed. Refer to the reference list as a guide to study specific areas.

We believe that you will find the questions, explanations, and format of the text to be of great assistance to you during your review. We wish you luck on the exam.

Jane S. Garofano

Acknowledgments

I acknowledge the National Certification Board for Therapeutic Massage and Bodywork (NCBTMB) for setting high standards for massage and bodyworkers nationally and giving me the opportunity to write questions to improve skills as well as professionalism.

A sincere thank you goes to Appleton & Lange's editorial staff, as well as Robin for the preparation and revision of the manuscript.

Practice Test Questions 1

DIRECTIONS: Each of the numbered items or incomplete statements in this chapter is followed by answers or completions of the statement. Select the **ONE** lettered answer or completion that is **BEST** in each case.

M   **1.** The sequences and directions of Swedish massage strokes are most adapted to which anatomical or physiological situation?
   A. Muscle attachments
   B. Subcutaneous adipose tissue
   C. Autonomic nervous system
   D. Lymph drainage and venous return

M   **2.** Which **BEST** describes the effects of massage therapy?
   A. Increased venous and lymph flow
   B. Increased venous, decreased arterial flow
   C. Decreased venous and lymph flow
   D. Decreased venous, increased lymph flow

M **3.** When massaging the thigh in the supine position, which is (are) involved?
   A. Hamstrings
   B. Quadriceps
   C. Gluteals
   D. Gastrocnemius

P **4.** Massage is contraindicated for which of the following conditions?
   A. High blood pressure
   B. Constipation
   C. Keloid scar
   D. Adhesions

AP **5.** The iliopsoas flexes the hip because of its insertion on the
   A. femur
   B. greater trochanter
   C. lesser trochanter
   D. iliac crest

AP **6.** The tricuspid valve is found between the
   A. right atrium and right ventricle
   B. left ventricle and aorta
   C. left ventricle and right ventricle
   D. right atrium and left atrium

B/E **7.** The purpose of a client-practitioner agreement is to
   A. develop clarity as to the nature of service
   B. protect from unrealistic expectations
   C. act as a consent reinforcement
   D. all of the above

AP **8.** Which structure supports the body in the sitting position?
   A. Sacrum
   B. Coccyx
   C. Ischial tuberosity
   D. L5

AP   **9.** Which statement is **TRUE** about Golgi tendon apparatus?
- **A.** Found in joint capsules
- **B.** Detects overall tension in tendon
- **C.** Originates in Purkinje fibers
- **D.** Activated by bagel reflex

AP   **10.** Which muscles are major adductors?
- **A.** Pectoralis and deltoid
- **B.** Pectoralis and latissimus dorsi
- **C.** Deltoid and latissimus dorsi
- **D.** Biceps and deltoids

P   **11.** Which muscle would be paralyzed if the sciatic nerve were severed?
- **A.** Trapezius
- **B.** Biceps femoris
- **C.** Gluteus maximus
- **D.** Erector spinae

AP   **12.** Which supplies the lower limbs?
- **A.** Dorsal primary rami
- **B.** Sciatic nerve
- **C.** Lumbosacral plexus
- **D.** Femoral nerve

AP   **13.** Which muscle laterally rotates, medially rotates, extends, and flexes?
- **A.** Gluteus maximus
- **B.** Gluteus minimus
- **C.** Gluteus medius
- **D.** Piriformis

M   **14.** In first aid for a choking victim, you want the victim to
- **A.** cough
- **B.** swallow
- **C.** vomit
- **D.** inhale

P   **15.** If massage is used in early stages of fracture healing, it should be given particularly on the area
        A. proximal to the actual site
        B. distal to the actual site
        C. medial to the actual site
        D. lateral to the actual site

AP   **16.** Which most accurately describes the meridian system?
        A. Energy pathway moving randomly through the body
        B. Energy pathway moving superficially
        C. Energy pathway that doesn't affect organs
        D. 12 meridians and 2 vessels are pathways in which energy moves toward the surface of the body, affecting organs

AP   **17.** A holistic bodywork that involves freeing the flow of energy through the body by using gentle rocking; the cradle; and an elbow milk is
        A. acupressure
        B. polarity therapy
        C. reflexology
        D. trigger point therapy

P   **18.** Which condition is present when there is an injury of the ulna nerve at the elbow?
        A. Inability to flex fingers fully
        B. Spasticity
        C. Flaccidity
        D. Spasms

AP   **19.** The Conception Vessel is the confluence of all the
        A. Yin channels
        B. Yang channels
        C. Qi energy
        D. five elements

P   **20.** To increase ROM, which is the most beneficial massage technique for a Colle's fracture directly out of a cast?
        A. Friction
        B. Rolling
        C. Tapotement
        D. Vibration

P   **21.** In treating a patient with kyphosis, which muscle or muscles should the massage therapist try to stretch and relax?
    A. Pectorals
    B. Rhomboids
    C. Erector spinae
    D. Trapezius

M   **22.** The massage therapist needs to wear gloves if
    A. there was no time to wash hands
    B. a client is embarrassed
    C. a client is infected with a contagious, transmittable disease
    D. his or her nails are too long

AP   **23.** The only joint in the upper body where the axial skeleton articulates with the appendicular skeleton is
    A. sternoclavicular
    B. glenohumeral
    C. sternoscapular
    D. scapularclavicular

AP   **24.** Which muscle adducts and medially rotates the femur at the hip?
    A. Gluteus medius
    B. Pectineus
    C. Quadratus femoris
    D. Tensor fascia latae

AP   **25.** Which muscle is closest to the sciatic nerve?
    A. Gracilis
    B. Piriformis
    C. Gluteus medius
    D. Pectineus

AP   **26.** Which is the most important element to combat skin infection?
    A. RBCs
    B. Platelets
    C. WBCs
    D. Fibrinogen

AP   **27.** Which muscle laterally rotates the femur at the hip joint?
- **A.** Pectineus
- **B.** Gluteus minimis
- **C.** Sartorius
- **D.** All of the above

AP   **28.** Which of the following is (are) **NOT** in the pelvic cavity?
- **A.** Kidneys
- **B.** Large intestines
- **C.** Ureters
- **D.** Urinary bladder

AP   **29.** Energy is stored in the muscle and liver for later use as
- **A.** glucose
- **B.** glycogen
- **C.** fructose
- **D.** pepsin

P   **30.** Which technique is recommended for rheumatoid arthritis?
- **A.** Effleurage
- **B.** Gentle friction
- **C.** Kneading
- **D.** Tapotement

M   **31.** A form of touch therapy in which the energy of the recipient is rebalanced, promoting health and healing, is called
- **A.** reflexology
- **B.** acupressure
- **C.** therapeutic touch
- **D.** lymph drainage

AP   **32.** Acupuncture, shiatsu, polarity, and reflexology are examples of
- **A.** energetic manipulation
- **B.** behavioral barometer
- **C.** reactive circuits
- **D.** systematic massage

M   **33.** Lymph massage procedures begin at the
   - **A.** tendons
   - **B.** left thoracic lymph duct
   - **C.** right thoracic lymph duct
   - **D.** immune system

M   **34.** Using neurophysical muscle reflexes to improve the functional mobility of the joints is called
   - **A.** kneading
   - **B.** NMT
   - **C.** muscle energy technique
   - **D.** stretching

M   **35.** A pregnant client should have pillows under her back when she is lying
   - **A.** on her side
   - **B.** supine
   - **C.** prone
   - **D.** upside down

AP   **36.** Which of the following is considered to be neutral on the pH scale?
   - **A.** Pure urine
   - **B.** Pure water
   - **C.** Pure blood
   - **D.** Pure saliva

M   **37.** A pre-event sports massage is basically a Swedish massage with the movements performed
   - **A.** precisely
   - **B.** using heat
   - **C.** slower
   - **D.** faster

M   **38.** Cross-fiber massage must be applied in which direction to the fibers?
   - **A.** Horizontal
   - **B.** At right angles
   - **C.** Triangular
   - **D.** Trapezoidal

M   **39.** MET helps to counteract
- **A.** soft tissue injury
- **B.** headache
- **C.** sprains
- **D.** muscle spasms

M   **40.** Cold applied for therapeutic purposes is called
- **A.** cryptology
- **B.** cryotherapy
- **C.** ignorance
- **D.** cool ice

M   **41.** The draping method that covers the entire body is called
- **A.** top-cover
- **B.** full-sheet
- **C.** diaper
- **D.** wrapping

M   **42.** The draping method that covers the table and wraps the client is called
- **A.** top-cover
- **B.** full-sheet
- **C.** diaper
- **D.** wrapping

M   **43.** At the start of a massage, the client is lying
- **A.** face up
- **B.** face down
- **C.** on his or her side
- **D.** any of the above

P   **44.** Massage can be beneficial for a headache with symptom(s) of
- **A.** sinus pressure
- **B.** vascular disruption
- **C.** toxins
- **D.** all of the above

M **45.** Most current massage styles are based on
   A. Swedish movements
   B. Swiss movements
   C. German movements
   D. Greek movements

P **46.** Thorough assessment of a client's condition reveals any
   A. lies
   B. weight gains
   C. credit gaps
   D. contraindications

B/E **47.** The letters SOAP refer to
   A. scale, office, access, plan
   B. subjective, open, area, parameter
   C. social, object, active, plan
   D. subjective, objective, assessment, plan

M **48.** Psychological benefits of massage include reduced tension and fatigue, calmer nerves, and
   A. therapeutics
   B. renewed energy
   C. improved circulation
   D. spasms

P **49.** Adhesion development and excessive scarring following trauma can be prevented or reduced with
   A. joint movements
   B. petrissage
   C. friction massage
   D. passive movements

M **50.** Friction, percussion, and vibration are techniques that
   A. stimulate
   B. relax
   C. strengthen
   D. weaken

P **51.** Techniques to avoid using on a pregnant client are heavy percussion and
   A. deep tissue massage
   B. tapotement
   C. petrissage
   D. lymph stimulation

AP **52.** A muscle contraction in which the distance between ends of the muscle changes is called
   A. isotonic
   B. resistant
   C. distal
   D. isometric

P **53.** Which of the following is a virus-induced mass produced by uncontrolled epithelial skin cell growth?
   A. Contusion
   B. Cyst
   C. Laceration
   D. Wart

M **54.** The kneading technique in which the practitioner attempts to grasp tissue and gently lift and spread it out is called
   A. fulling
   B. pulling
   C. spreading
   D. nudging

M **55.** Pressing one superficial layer of tissue against a deeper layer of tissue in order to flatten the deeper layer is called
   A. rolling
   B. spreading
   C. friction
   D. ironing

AP **56.** Normal body temperature is (in degrees Fahrenheit, °F)
   A. 97.3
   B. 98.6
   C. 99.2
   D. 101.1

AP 57. The movements at synovial joints include flexion/extension, abduction/adduction, and
    A. rotation
    B. isolation
    C. dynamics
    D. pivot

B/E 58. Many massage therapists are confronted with obstacles that diminish the drive and motivation of a new business such as
    A. burnout
    B. start-up costs
    C. lack of advertising knowledge
    D. all of the above

AP 59. The term "dorsal" means
    A. next to
    B. in back of
    C. in front of
    D. middle

M 60. Nerve trunks and centers are sometimes chosen as sites for the application of
    A. rolling
    B. rocking
    C. pressure
    D. vibration

AP 61. The finger pressure massage method called *shiatsu* is
    A. Japanese
    B. Chinese
    C. German
    D. French

M 62. A bath with a temperature of 85°F to 95°F is considered
    A. cool
    B. cold
    C. tepid
    D. hot

M   **63.** Warm baths should be followed by a (an)
      A. cool shower
      B. whirlpool
      C. salt bath
      D. ice pack

AP   **64.** Which of the following is **NOT** in the appendicular skeleton?
      A. Coccyx
      B. Fibula
      C. Humerus
      D. Hyoid

M   **65.** The source of pain can be pinpointed through
      A. palpation
      B. hard end feel
      C. inert tissues
      D. knuckling

M   **66.** The procedure that uses a bouncing movement to improve the flow of lymph through the entire system is called lymphatic
      A. bounce
      B. sway
      C. purging
      D. pump manipulation

M   **67.** The attempt to bring the structure of the body into alignment around a central axis is called
      A. structural integration
      B. trauma
      C. alignment
      D. adjustment

M   **68.** Realignment of muscular and connective tissue and reshaping the body's physical posture is called
      A. adjustment
      B. centering
      C. Rolfing
      D. posturing

M **69.** A hyperirritable spot that is painful when compressed is called a (an)
   A. trigger point
   B. pain point
   C. ampule
   D. Rolfing

M **70.** Better flexibility is the result of
   A. sustained stretching
   B. ballistic stretching
   C. weight lifting
   D. bicycling

P **71.** Relieving soreness, tension, and stiffness with massage can benefit the
   A. muscular system
   B. skeletal system
   C. respiratory system
   D. excretory system

P **72.** In order to evaluate projected pain it is necessary to know the
   A. portion of the brain involved
   B. proximal nerve that is compressed
   C. distal nerve that is compressed
   D. none of the above

P **73.** Cirrhosis of the liver can benefit from massage for
   A. toxemia
   B. stress reduction
   C. drug withdrawal
   D. B and C

M **74.** Linens should be washed
   A. when very dirty
   B. monthly
   C. after each use
   D. twice monthly

P   **75.** A sprain with extensive swelling is caused by a twist of the
- **A.** muscle
- **B.** wrist
- **C.** joint
- **D.** tendon

P   **76.** Injuries that have a gradual onset or reoccur often are called
- **A.** sprains
- **B.** occupational
- **C.** acute
- **D.** chronic

AP   **77.** Which of the following factors contribute to muscle fatigue?
- **A.** Insufficient oxygen
- **B.** Depletion of glycogen
- **C.** Lactic acid buildup
- **D.** All of the above

AP   **78.** A sudden involuntary contraction of a muscle is called a (an)
- **A.** levator
- **B.** proximal
- **C.** isometric
- **D.** spasm

P   **79.** A muscle strain that involves a partial tear of 10% to 50% of the muscle fibers is classified as
- **A.** Grade I
- **B.** Grade II
- **C.** Grade III
- **D.** parietal

AP   **80.** Which type of lever is characterized as having the fulcrum between the effort and resistance? An example is the head resting on the vertebral column.
- **A.** First class
- **B.** Second class
- **C.** Third class
- **D.** Fourth class

P

81. A muscle that has been injured to the point of subacute stage needs how many days to recover?

    A. 1–2
    B. 2–3
    C. 3–5
    D. 5–7

M

82. A centering exercise in which you turn your arm in a circle is called

    A. the wheel
    B. grinding corn
    C. grounding
    D. centering

AP

83. Actively moving muscles helps prevent loss of

    A. body fat
    B. brain tissue
    C. tone and strength
    D. teeth

P

84. Terminology related to massage is derived from which profession?

    A. Cosmetology
    B. Health and medicine
    C. Psychiatry
    D. Athletics

B/E

85. If a client's condition is outside the massage technician's scope of practice, the technician should

    A. schedule extra sessions
    B. refer the client to the proper professional
    C. take more training
    D. read textbooks

B/E

86. Many cities have massage ordinances to

    A. promote business
    B. raise money
    C. keep clerks employed
    D. curb illegal activities

AP **87.** Which facial muscle inserts into the mandible, angles of the mouth, and skin of the lower face?
- **A.** Buccinator
- **B.** Depressor labii inferior
- **C.** Levator labii superioris
- **D.** Platysma

AP **88.** The branch of biology concerned with the microscopic structure of living tissues is
- **A.** physiology
- **B.** histology
- **C.** anatomy
- **D.** pathology

AP **89.** Anabolism and catabolism are closely regulated to maintain
- **A.** prophase
- **B.** enzymes
- **C.** amitosis
- **D.** homeostasis

M **90.** According to Dolores Krieger, therapeutic touch is most effective on
- **A.** fluid and electrolytes
- **B.** ANS
- **C.** lymphatic and circulatory problems
- **D.** all of the above

B/E **91.** A relaxing atmosphere for massage may be created with
- **A.** clothing
- **B.** music
- **C.** wall coverings
- **D.** carpet

B/E **92.** Reviewing records before a client's visit refreshes your memory and gains the client's
- **A.** muscle aches
- **B.** billing information
- **C.** trust
- **D.** extra treatments

B/E   **93.** All client information should be considered
- **A.** nonessential
- **B.** lifesaving
- **C.** boring
- **D.** confidential

M   **94.** Using too much deep pressure causes the muscles to
- **A.** have pain
- **B.** go limp
- **C.** relax
- **D.** cramp

AP   **95.** What is the spinal nerve contribution that composes the brachial plexus?
- **A.** C_1–C_4; T_1
- **B.** C_5–C_8; T_1
- **C.** C_7–C_8; T_1
- **D.** T_2–T_{12}; L_1

AP   **96.** Cardiac muscle tissue occurs only in the
- **A.** liver
- **B.** stomach
- **C.** heart
- **D.** mouth

P   **97.** The part of the brain that projects the pain back to the stimulated area is the
- **A.** cerebral cortex
- **B.** corpus callosum
- **C.** thalamus
- **D.** hypothalamus

AP   **98.** In anatomy, the sagittal plane divides the body into left and right parts by an imaginary line running
- **A.** vertically
- **B.** horizontally
- **C.** diagonally
- **D.** circularly

P **99.** Which nerve is affected in carpal tunnel syndrome?
   A. Axillary
   B. Median
   C. Medial pectoral
   D. Radial

P **100.** Light massage can, over time, restore energy to a client suffering from
   A. fatigue
   B. shingles
   C. varicose veins
   D. acne

M **101.** The general effects of percussion movements are to tone the muscles by
   A. vibration
   B. friction
   C. kneading
   D. hacking, cupping, slapping, beating

AP **102.** Which of the following muscles are forearm flexors at the elbow joint?
   A. Biceps brachii, brachialis, triceps brachii
   B. Brachioradialis, anconeus, pronator quadratus
   C. Supinator, brachialis, biceps brachii
   D. Brachialis, brachioradialis, biceps brachii

AP **103.** Aligning major body segments through manipulation of connective tissue is the
   A. Rolfing method
   B. Trager method
   C. Palmer method
   D. Reflexology method

M **104.** The idea that stimulation of particular body points affects other areas is called
   A. chiropractic
   B. reflexology
   C. Rolfing
   D. touching

AP **105.** Applied kinesiology methods are designed to relieve stress on muscles and
A. joints
B. bones
C. ligaments
D. internal organs

AP **106.** A type of specialized kinesiology used to evaluate energetic imbalances in the body is called
A. SMB
B. precision muscle testing
C. orthobionomy
D. tender point

AP **107.** The traditional Chinese medical practice in which the skin is punctured with needles is called
A. reflexology
B. sewing
C. acupuncture
D. chop sticks

P **108.** The popliteal fossa is an endangerment site because of
A. lymph nodes
B. tibial and peroneal nerves
C. median cubital vein
D. kidney

P **109.** To reduce adhesions and fibrosis, which of the following movements is used?
A. Cross-fiber friction
B. Wringing
C. Pressing
D. Squeezing

AP **110.** Which of the following does not flex the wrist?
A. Flexor carpi radialis
B. Flexor carpi ulnaris
C. Pronator quadratus
D. Palmaris longus

M **111.** The stance in which both feet are placed perpendicular to the edge of the table is called the
   A. archer
   B. horse
   C. moose
   D. stirrup

P **112.** Massage interfaces with the effects of many medications and therefore it is important to reference drugs in the
   A. Gray's Anatomy
   B. Physicians Desk Reference
   C. Webster's dictionary
   D. medical dictionary

P **113.** Massage therapists should be able to assess the effects of medications that alter muscle tone, cardiovascular function, anti-inflammatory as well as
   A. anticoagulants
   B. personality
   C. analgesics
   D. all of the above

M **114.** The ability to carry on an activity over a prolonged period of time and resist fatigue is called
   A. strength
   B. muscle bulk
   C. endurance
   D. exercise

P **115.** Pathogenic organisms cause the development of many disease processes and include
   A. virus and bacteria
   B. fungi
   C. protozoa and metazoa worms
   D. all of the above

P **116.** Severe strain of the trapezius and deltoid muscles is called
   A. racquetball shoulder
   B. tennis elbow
   C. skier's snap
   D. bowler's break

P   **117.** Overstretching of the gracilis and adductor muscle on the inner thigh results from
- **A.** soccer
- **B.** tennis
- **C.** horseback riding
- **D.** bowling

P   **118.** The client may react to pain with
- **A.** fear and anxiety
- **B.** ischemic response
- **C.** active movement
- **D.** passive movement

P   **119.** Severe varicose veins is a (an) _____ for massage.
- **A.** Indication
- **B.** Circulation
- **C.** Embolus
- **D.** Contraindication

AP   **120.** Which of the following is **NOT** a hamstring muscle?
- **A.** Adductor magnus
- **B.** Biceps femoris
- **C.** Semimembranosus
- **D.** Semitendinosus

AP   **121.** Which is **NOT** part of the sternum?
- **A.** Styloid process
- **B.** Manubrium
- **C.** Xiphoid process
- **D.** Gladiolus

AP   **122.** What forms the outer layer of the anterior and lateral abdominal wall?
- **A.** Rectus abdominis
- **B.** Transversalis
- **C.** Serratus anterior
- **D.** External oblique

AP **123.** The primary flexor of the distal phalanges of the fingers is
    A. flexor carpi ulnaris
    B. pollices longus
    C. flexor digitorum profundus
    D. flexor carpi radialis

AP **124.** The body's normal posture has what type of contraction?
    A. Tetanic
    B. Isotonic
    C. Isometric
    D. Tonus

AP **125.** Inguinal nodes serve the purpose of draining lymph from the
    A. arm
    B. lower neck
    C. neck
    D. leg

M **126.** Joint mobilizationis a passive movement that can be integrated into a massage routine, for example
    A. pulling
    B. friction
    C. stretching to ROM limit
    D. tapotement

AP **127.** The energy for the stomach meridian is most effective from
    A. 7 a.m. to 9 a.m.
    B. 7 p.m. to 9 p.m.
    C. 3 a.m. to 5 a.m.
    D. 3 p.m. to 5 p.m.

AP **128.** The energy for the spleen meridian is most effective from
    A. 7 a.m. to 9 a.m.
    B. 7 p.m. to 9 p.m.
    C. 9 a.m. to 11 a.m.
    D. 11 p.m. to 1 a.m.

P   **129.** Sciatic nerve damage diminishes ability to
  A. flex the hip
  B. flex the knee
  C. adduct the hip
  D. abduct the hip

P   **130.** Swelling of one entire leg is usually caused by pathology in
  A. heart muscle
  B. a blood vessel
  C. kidney
  D. liver

P   **131.** In a patient with subdeltoid bursitis, the pain is worse if the arm is
  A. abducted
  B. adducted
  C. hyperextended
  D. laterally rotated

M   **132.** Deep strokes and kneading techniques can cause an increase in
  A. vasoconstriction
  B. blood flow
  C. diastolic arterial pressure
  D. systolic arterial pressure

P   **133.** Arthritis is a (an)
  A. vitamin A deficiency
  B. vitamin C deficiency
  C. inflammation of the joints
  D. bone fracture

M   **134.** What **BEST** describes the technique of Rolfing?
  A. Reflex zone therapy
  B. German massage
  C. Structural integration
  D. Connective tissue massage

AP   135. The cerebellum
    A. functions to maintain proper posture and equilibrium
    B. receives input from the motor cortex and basal ganglia
    C. receives input from proprioceptors in joints and muscles
    D. has all of the above characteristics

AP   136. Which body substance is composed primarily of dense fibrous tissue?
    A. Muscle
    B. Nerve tissue
    C. Tendon
    D. Bone

AP   137. The membrane that surrounds the shaft of a long bone is the
    A. synovial membrane
    B. bursae
    C. periosteum
    D. peritoneum

AP   138. Manipulation of the occipital regions of the neck primarily affects
    A. HT and BL meridians
    B. CO and KI meridians
    C. BL and GB meridians
    D. ST and SP meridians

P   139. Facial paralysis can be due to a lesion in which cranial nerve?
    A. III
    B. VI
    C. VII
    D. VIII

P   140. In chronic swelling around the patella, what massage technique do you use on the thigh?
    A. Kneading of the thigh
    B. Friction of the knee
    C. Effleurage proximal to knee
    D. Effleurage distal to knee

AP   **141.** Which muscle elevates and depresses the scapula?
     A. Trapezius
     B. Latissimus dorsi
     C. Rhomboids
     D. All of the above

AP   **142.** With the elbow flexed, which muscle supinates the palm?
     A. Pronator
     B. Supinator
     C. Quadrator
     D. Brachialis

AP   **143.** Which of the following is paired correctly?
     A. Chemoreceptors–detect smell and taste
     B. Mechanoreceptors–detect temperature
     C. Nociceptors–detect light
     D. Photoreceptors–detect stretching

P   **144.** Inflammation of the walls of the vein is called
     A. aneurysm
     B. phlebitis
     C. varicose vein
     D. atherosclerosis

P   **145.** When treating swelling due to a dislocated knee, which technique is valuable?
     A. Effleurage
     B. Kneading
     C. Tapotement
     D. Friction

M   **146.** Deep friction massage works **BEST** if it is applied
     A. directly over problem area
     B. proximal to problem area
     C. distal to problem area
     D. around the problem area

M   **147.** The cupping technique is best suited for
   - **A.** acute bronchitis
   - **B.** cancer of the lungs
   - **C.** bronchiectasis
   - **D.** acute tracheitis

P   **148.** Most of the stress and pain that responds to therapeutic massage involve the
   - **A.** circulatory and nervous system
   - **B.** nervous and endocrine systems
   - **C.** muscle system
   - **D.** none of the above

AP   **149.** The last step in clot formation is
   - **A.** prothrombin to thrombin
   - **B.** fibrinogen to fibrin
   - **C.** platelet formation
   - **D.** tissue trauma

AP   **150.** The exchange of O_2 and CO_2 takes place in
   - **A.** alveoli
   - **B.** bronchi
   - **C.** bronchioles
   - **D.** pleural cavity

Practice Test Questions 1

Answers and Discussion

1. **(D)**   The principle of Swedish massage is always to massage toward the heart in order to move venous blood and lymph back to the thoracic duct and right atrium. *(Ref. 2, p. 250)*

2. **(A)**   All circulation is improved by massage of muscles stimulating blood back to the heart and circulating lymph through elimination organs. *(Ref. 2, p. 247)*

3. **(B)**   The quadriceps are the muscles of the anterior thigh when in the supine position. *(Ref. 2, p. 409)*

4. **(A)**   High blood pressure is a contraindicator due to the increased pressure exerted on the walls of the arteries. *(Ref. 2, p. 258)*

5. **(C)**   The action of the iliopsoas is to flex the hip up, and the psoas is inserted on the lesser trochanter of the femur to accomplish this action. *(Ref. 7, p. 95)*

6. **(A)**   The blood flow from the right atrium to the right ventricle is through the tricuspid valve to keep the blood flowing in one direction. *(Ref. 2, p. 165)*

7. **(D)**   A client-practitioner agreement and policy statement are important to inform the client and protect the therapist. *(Ref. 11, p. 170)*

8. (C) The ischial tuberosity is the posterior portion of the ramus of the ischium, where the bodyweight is supported. *(Ref. 7, p. 90)*

9. (B) The golgi tendon organ is a proprioceptor. Proprioceptors are multibranched sensory nerve endings in tendons that measure tension in the muscle. *(Ref. 2, p. 202)*

10. (B) Adductor muscles of the upper body that bring the arms toward the body include the pectoralis major and latissimus dorsi. *(Ref. 2, p. 126)*

11. (B) The biceps femoris would be paralyzed if the sciatic nerve were severed, since it controls the flexion of the posterior thigh and leg. *(Ref. 2, p. 210; Ref. 3, p. 149)*

12. (C) The lumbosacral plexus include all the spinal nerves exit from L1 to L5 and the sacral vertebrae supplying the lower limbs. *(Ref. 3, p. 150)*

13. (C) The lateral gluteus medius contributes many movements of the hip and lower limbs, including rotation and flexion. *(Ref. 7, p. 99)*

14. (A) If choking, a victim should cough first to remove any object. *(Ref. 1, pp. 108–110)*

15. (A) Massage to the proximal area of a fracture promotes healing by stimulating circulation. *(Ref. 2, p. 99)*

16. (D) The 12 bilateral meridians in the body conduct energy along pathways that are related to organs and the chi (energy). *(Ref. 5, p. 135)*

17. (B) Polarity supports health and healing by releasing obstructions using the cradle, elbow milk, and rocking. *(Ref. 5, p. 210)*

18. (C) Sensation-motion is eliminated from the elbow to the fingers due to nerve damage. *(Ref. 2, p. 209)*

19. **(A)** All the Yin channels meet with the deep and superficial pathways of the Conception Vessels at CV1 to CV24. *(Ref. 12, p. 92)*

20. **(A)** Friction at the wrist helps to mobilize the joint and increase flexibility in order to restore full range of motion. *(Ref. 2, pp. 591–594)*

21. **(A)** Massage to the pectorals of the chest, by stretching and relaxing, can aid the exaggerated convex curve of the thoracic spine. *(Ref. 2, p. 102)*

22. **(C)** In special situations the therapist should wear gloves to prevent the spread of a contagious disease. *(Ref. 11, p. 113)*

23. **(A)** The sternum of the rib cage of the axial skeleton articulates with the clavicle bone, which is part of the appendicular skeleton. *(Ref. 3, p. 125)*

24. **(B)** The pectineus, the uppermost medial thigh muscle attached to the pubis and femur, is for rotation and adduction. *(Ref. 2, p. 138; Ref. 7, p. 102)*

25. **(B)** The piriformis muscle is very close to the sciatic nerve as its origin is on the greater sciatic notch, and is innervated at L5 and S1 at the sacral plexus. *(Ref. 2, p. 139)*

26. **(C)** The white blood cells fight any infection by engulfing and digesting bacteria and producing antibodies for protection from disease organisms. *(Ref. 2, p. 173)*

27. **(C)** The sartorius inserts on the greater trochanter of the femur in order to provide lateral rotation at the hip. *(Ref. 2, p. 139)*

28. **(A)** The kidneys lie in the abdominal cavity at T12 vertebra. *(Ref. 8, p. 18)*

29. **(B)** Glycogen is converted from glucose and stored in the liver for later use as a source of energy. *(Ref. 8, p. 251)*

30. **(B)** Gentle friction helps to milk out body fluids from the inflamed joint. It also softens the massed ground substance between layers of tissue. *(Ref. 2, pp. 100, 318)*

31. **(C)** Therapeutic touch is a technique of centering and placing the hands in the recipient's energy field to detect a break in energy flow. *(Ref. 5, p. 350)*

32. **(A)** There is a force, or vibration, that, when smooth, results in good health. Techniques detect imbalance in the force and through energetic manipulation regain homeostasis. *(Ref. 2, p. 573; Ref. 4, p. 62)*

33. **(C)** Lymph massage starts at the right side of the body to drain into the right thoracic lymph duct. Both sides should not be done at the same time. *(Ref. 2, p. 545)*

34. **(C)** MET uses active muscle constriction followed by relaxation and passive stretching to increase ROM. *(Ref. 2, p. 554)*

35. **(B)** Pillows under the back and knees are more comfortable for a pregnant woman. *(Ref. 2, p. 539)*

36. **(B)** Water is the standard pH of 7. *(Ref. 8, p. 40)*

37. **(D)** A pre-event sports massage is a faster, shorter, and more intense technique to prepare the athlete's body for better performance. *(Ref. 2, pp. 515–523)*

38. **(B)** For cross-fiber massage to be effective on the muscle fibers, application must be at a right angle to spread them apart. *(Ref. 5, p. 84)*

39. **(D)** The muscle energy tissue (MET) helps to contract a target muscle without spasm by applying more resistance than the force of the contraction. *(Ref. 2, p. 554)*

40. **(B)** Cryotherapy is a cold therapy to eliminate pain and allow for massage treatment. *(Ref. 2, p. 464)*

41. **(A)** A top-cover allows the client to be fully covered by a sheet as well as using a sheet to cover the table. *(Ref. 2, p. 356)*

42. **(B)**   The client can be draped using the sheet on the table by lifting it up over the body. *(Ref. 2, p. 356)*

43. **(D)**   In preparation for body massage, assist the client onto the table and into a supine (face up) or prone position. *(Ref. 5, p. 93)*

44. **(D)**   Massage can benefit a pain or dull ache in the head or neck causing sinus pressure, muscle tension, release of toxins, or vascular disruption. *(Ref. 11, p. 402)*

45. **(A)**   Swedish massage is classified as using the fundamental manipulation of massage used today. Most treatments combine one or more of these movements. *(Ref. 2, p. 305)*

46. **(D)**   Contraindications should be revealed when the client's history is taken. They can include past/present diseases, disorders, and psychological problems. *(Ref. 2, pp. 253–259)*

47. **(D)**   SOAP charting is an efficient, effective way to document all types of healthcare treatment through a subjective and objective assessment and plan for the client. *(Ref. 14, p. 7)*

48. **(B)**   There is a renewed sense of energy as a result of promoting relaxation and relieving fatigue and tension through massage. *(Ref. 2, p. 247)*

49. **(C)**   Adhesions and scarring can be relieved by regular friction massage. Constrictions can be reduced as the muscle tissue heals. *(Ref. 2, p. 253)*

50. **(A)**   The muscle is stimulated by friction, percussion, and vibration by moving superficial layers against deeper muscle layers of tissue. *(Ref. 2, p. 318)*

51. **(A)**   Massage during pregnancy should be soothing and relaxing, never deep tissue massage or abdominal kneading or deep abdominal massage. *(Ref. 2, p. 260)*

52. **(A)**   When parts of the body move in the action, the contraction is isotonic. *(Ref. 2, p. 114)*

53. (D) Warts are known to be caused by viruses causing the skin to grow in an uncontrolled fashion. *(Ref. 8, p. 142)*

54. (A) Techniques of the kneading massage include squeezing, pressing, lifting, or fulling the skin. *(Ref. 2, p. 307)*

55. (C) Friction strokes include the pressure of one layer of tissue (or skin) over the deeper layer to improve blood flow to area. *(Ref. 2, p. 318)*

56. (B) The body is stabilized at a temperature of 98.6°F. Both water and illness affect this temperature. *(Ref. 2, p. 470)*

57. (A) The movement of bones occurring at synovial joint is called range of motion, and includes flexion, adduction, and rotation. *(Ref. 3, p. 34)*

58. (D) Many massage therapists have difficulty and fail in their new business due to burnout, lack of funds, or lack of marketing skills. *(Ref. 11, pp. 151–155)*

59. (B) The directional term that means in the back of is "dorsal" or "posterior." *(Ref. 3, p. 2)*

60. (D) Vibration treatment follows the path of the nerve: gentle, rhythmical, and fine vibration to the nerve trunk. *(Ref. 5, pp. 91–92)*

61. (A) The Japanese word *shiatsu* means pressure of the fingers: *shi* (finger) and *atsu* (pressure). *(Ref. 2, p. 567)*

62. (C) A tepid (slightly warm) bath is soothing and relaxing, good for nervous and excited people. *(Ref. 2, p. 473)*

63. (A) A cool shower after a warm bath stimulates nerves and awakens the functional activity of body cells. *(Ref. 2, p. 473)*

64. (D) The axial skeleton contains the skull, vertebrae, ribs, and hyoid bone. *(Ref. 8, p. 168)*

65. (A) Palpation is the primary source of assessing pain on hypersensitive points and areas by an objective or subjective approach of touch. *(Ref. 2, p. 439)*

66. **(D)** The lymphatic pump manipulation enhances the flow of lymph and can be done with the lymph drainage massage. Pressure and pumping on the chest is done, 150 bounces per minute, to expel the breath. *(Ref. 2, p. 547)*

67. **(A)** Structural integration is done by manipulating the fascia of the structural muscles resulting from poor posture and binding of connective tissue. *(Ref. 2, p. 548)*

68. **(C)** Rolfing is a method of structural integration intended to correctly align the spine and body segments by the use of heavy pressure of knuckles, fist, or elbow into the muscle and connective tissue. *(Ref. 2, p. 549)*

69. **(A)** Palpating muscles effectively locates trigger points that are associated with soft tissue pain and dysfunction. *(Ref. 2, p. 439)*

70. **(A)** The mechanical effect of massage is the stretching of superficial tissue, which encourages better flexibility. *(Ref. 5, p. 24)*

71. **(A)** Massage benefits the muscle system and joints that are sore due to tension and stiffness. The circulation is improved and the muscles become more supple. *(Ref. 2, p. 252)*

72. **(B)** Pain is perceived in the tissue supplied by the proximal nerve to the location. *(Ref. 11, p. 93)*

73. **(D)** Massage is indicated for stress and drug withdrawal if cirrhosis of the liver is diagnosed. *(Ref. 11, p. 409)*

74. **(C)** All towels and linens should be cleaned after each use to prevent a spread of infection. *(Ref. 2, p. 355)*

75. **(C)** An injury to a joint with a tearing or stretching of the ligament and swelling is considered a severe sprain. *(Ref. 2, p. 100)*

76. **(D)** Chronic injuries occur over time or are longlasting, and they can benefit from gentle massage depending on the injury. *(Ref. 2, p. 508)*

77. (D) Many factors contribute to muscle fatigue, including a lactic acid buildup and depletion of oxygen, calcium, and glycogen. *(Ref. 8, p. 252)*

78. (D) A muscle spasm is a sudden involuntary contraction of the muscle when the nerve to the muscle is irritated. *(Ref. 2, p. 120)*

79. (B) Grade II muscle strain has pain and some loss of function and some tissue bleeding. *(Ref. 2, p. 120)*

80. (A) The first-class lever is like a seesaw as the head is resting on the vertebrae. When the head is raised the facial area is in resistance. The fulcrum is between the effort and resistance. *(Ref. 8, p. 271)*

81. (B) After the subacute stage, the swelling and inflammation have subsided and the healing process has begun. Allow 2–3 days for recovery from the injury. *(Ref. 2, p. 522)*

82. (A) The wheel is a good centering exercise that involves shifting body weight forward and backward, rotating the hand around in a circle. *(Ref. 2, p. 343)*

83. (C) Muscle tone is present in healthy muscles; exercise and massage help to improve this condition. *(Ref. 2, p. 113)*

84. (B) Health and medicine were the roots of massage remedial treatment for disease as well as physical therapy for rehabilitation. *(Ref. 2, p. 12)*

85. (B) A client should always be referred to another health practitioner if the treatment required goes beyond massage. *(Ref. 2, p. 295)*

86. (D) To curb illegal massage activities, many cities have ordinances regulating practitioners. *(Ref. 2, p. 21)*

87. (D) The platysma is the superficial muscle of the face that moves the lip downward and backward by inserting on the mandible. *(Ref. 8, p. 279)*

88. (B) Histology is the microscopic structure of the tissues. *(Ref. 2, p. 35)*

89. (D) Homeostasis is regulated by metabolism maintaining a normal, stable internal environment. *(Ref. 2, p. 55)*

90. (D) Therapeutic touch, developed by Dolores Krieger, benefits fluid and electrolyte levels, the ANS, and lymphatic and circulatory problems. *(Ref. 5, p. 350)*

91. (B) Using music that is soft and soothing can enhance a relaxing massage. *(Ref. 2, p. 272)*

92. (C) Reviewing accurate records prior to massage establishes confidence and trust on the part of the client. *(Ref. 2, p. 302)*

93. (D) All personal information regarding a client should be kept in a secure place and confidential. *(Ref. 2, p. 302)*

94. (A) Deep pressure techniques such as Rolfing must be done with caution to avoid too much pain. *(Ref. 2, p. 309)*

95. (B) The brachial plexus contributes spinal nerves through C_5–C_8 and T_1 only. *(Ref. 8, p. 393)*

96. (C) There are three types of muscle tissue: skeletal, smooth, and cardiac. Only cardiac muscle occurs in the heart. *(Ref. 2, p. 105)*

97. (B) The liquid connective tissue of the body is the blood, consisting of cells and plasma. *(Ref. 8, p. 118)*

98. (A) The cerebral cortex locates the origin of pain related to past experiences back to the stimulated area. *(Ref. 11, p. 95)*

99. (B) The median nerve of the brachial plexus is injured in carpal tunnel syndrome by the compression of the nerve through the carpal tunnel. *(Ref. 8, p. 394)*

100. (A) A benefit of massage is to increase circulation and stimulate muscles, thus relieving fatigue. *(Ref. 2, p. 247)*

101. (D) A rapid striking motion—using different amounts of force and hand positions such as hacking, cupping, or slapping—tones the muscles. *(Ref. 2, pp. 323–324)*

102. (D) The flexors at the elbow joint include the brachialis, brachioradialis, and biceps brachii. These muscles all help to flex the forearm. *(Ref. 8, p. 308)*

103. (A) The fascia can be manipulated through the Rolfing method. *(Ref. 2, p. 16)*

104. (B) Organs and functions of the body can be affected by pressing reflex zones on the hands and feet. The technique is reflexology. *(Ref. 2, p. 572; Ref. 5, p. 255)*

105. (D) The internal organs can be relieved through the process of applied kinesiology, that is, the principles of anatomy in relation to human movement. *(Ref. 2, p. 17)*

106. (B) Precision muscle testing is used to evaluate the energy imbalance and to determine which remedies will work best for an individual. *(Ref. 2, p. 560)*

107. (C) Acupuncture is a type of acupressure on points throughout the body. *(Ref. 5, p. 133)*

108. (B) Endangerment sites on the body represent areas that can be injured due to exposure of vessels, organs, and nerves to deep massage. The tibial and peroneal nerve are endangered in the fossa of the knee. *(Ref. 2, p. 265)*

109. (A) Cross-fiber friction is the best stroke to prevent or reduce adhesions, and fibrosis manipulation moves fibers apart from each other. *(Ref. 2, p. 557)*

110. (C) The pronator quadratus is responsible for pronating the forearm and wrist. *(Ref. 8, p. 308)*

111. (B) The foot positions in posture and stances aid balance and allow a more direct delivery of massage strokes. The horse is a common one in which both feet are placed perpendicular to the table. *(Ref. 2, p. 336)*

112. **(B)** The Physicians Desk Reference helps therapists to recognize the indications and contraindications to a client's medication. *(Ref. 11, p. 99)*

113. **(D)** Because many medications have side effects, it is important to be familiar with the various types that affect different areas of the body and mind. *(Ref. 11, p. 99)*

114. **(C)** Endurance is a function of resisting fatigue and is related to the development of the cardiovascular system. *(Ref. 2, p. 588)*

115. **(D)** Many viruses, bacteria, protozoa, and worms cause pathogenic diseases, which must be prevented by use of sanitary conditions or contraindicated for massage. *(Ref. 11, p. 109)*

116. **(A)** The shoulder and back muscles can be strained from sports such as racquet ball and tennis. *(Ref. 2, p. 532)*

117. **(C)** The gracilis and adductor muscles are stretched by the action of horseback riding. *(Ref. 7, p. 109)*

118. **(A)** Depending on the level of pain and experience related to an injury, a client's fear and anxiety can vary. *(Ref. 2, p. 38)*

119. **(D)** If a client has varicose veins, it is not recommended to apply massage. This is a contraindication. *(Ref. 2, pp. 256–257)*

120. **(A)** The hamstring muscles of the posterior thigh include the biceps femoris, semimembranosus, and semitendinosus. The adductors do not flex. *(Ref. 8, p. 330)*

121. **(A)** The styloid process is not a part of the sternum; it is part of the radius and ulna bone. *(Ref. 3, p. 24)*

122. **(D)** Four muscles form the abdominal wall, with the external oblique being the most superficial. *(Ref. 3, p. 43)*

123. **(C)** The distal phalanges are flexed by the flexor digitorum profundus. *(Ref. 7, p. 71)*

124. **(D)** When the muscles are stationary or at rest, they possess a firm condition called muscle tone. *(Ref. 2, p. 113)*

125. **(D)** The body has regional lymph nodes for drainage. The inguinal nodes drain the legs at the groin. *(Ref. 2, p. 185)*

126. **(C)** Stretching is used to mobilize and increase the flexibility at the joint as it elongates the muscle and connective tissue. *(Ref. 5, p. 107)*

127. **(A)** The energy for the stomach meridian is most effective from 7 a.m. to 9 a.m. *(Ref. 5, p. 173)*

128. **(C)** The energy for the spleen meridian is most effective from 9 a.m. to 11 a.m. *(Ref. 5, p. 173)*

129. **(B)** The sciatic nerve innervates the leg, and damage can limit the mobility of knee flexing. *(Ref. 2, pp. 110, 142)*

130. **(B)** Edema, or swelling, can result from phlebitis, a blockage in the venous system. *(Ref. 2, p. 170)*

131. **(A)** Joint mobility, especially abduction, is limited at the bursae due to trauma or repeated irritation. *(Ref. 2, p. 101)*

132. **(B)** Any deep pressure strokes stimulate the circulation and therefore blood flow. *(Ref. 2, p. 253)*

133. **(C)** An inflammatory condition of the joints and bone damage is characteristic of arthritis. *(Ref. 2, p. 101)*

134. **(C)** Rolfing aligns the major body segments through fascia manipulation to establish structural integration. *(Ref. 2, p. 16)*

135. **(D)** The cerebellum in the brain is responsible for posture and equilibrium, and receives input from the motor cortex and basal ganglia as well as the proprioceptor. *(Ref. 8, p. 418)*

136. **(C)** The tendons that attach muscle to bone are fibrous connective tissue. *(Ref. 2, p. 59; Ref. 3, p.6)*

137. **(C)** Anatomically the structure of a bone has a membrane over the compact bone called the periosteum. *(Ref. 2, p. 58)*

138. (C) Massaging the bladder and gall bladder meridians affects the heart and neck muscles. *(Ref. 2, p. 566)*

139. (C) The nerve that controls facial muscles is number VII and would affect any facial paralysis. *(Ref. 2, p. 195)*

140. (C) Effleurage is the best massage technique for moving fluid from the knee and back to the heart and lymphatic ducts. *(Ref. 5, p. 102)*

141. (A) The trapezius muscle touches the scapula and functions in elevating and depressing shoulders. *(Ref. 7, p. 18)*

142. (B) The supinator muscle is responsible for the palm of the hand in supination. *(Ref. 7, p. 55)*

143. (A) The senses of smell and taste are both classified as chemoreceptors in the nose and mouth. *(Ref. 8, p. 445)*

144. (B) Pain, swelling, and inflammation are characteristic of phlebitis of the veins. *(Ref. 2, p. 256)*

145. (A) Effleurage around swelling is advantageous for knee injuries. Use the tips of fingers for knee stress points. *(Ref. 2, p. 528)*

146. (D) The best treatment around a problem area for swelling or pain is deep friction massage. *(Ref. 2, p. 529)*

147. (C) Congestive lung conditions are treated with the cupping technique of percussion. *(Ref. 2, p. 324)*

148. (B) The nervous and endocrine systems are responsible for most stress patterns that can be relieved by disrupting the signals of the sensory receptors. *(Ref. 11, p. 122)*

149. (B) The protein fibrin is the end product of a clot formation. *(Ref. 2, p. 173)*

150. (A) The alveoli are the microscopic air sacs that exchange gases with the blood capillaries of the lungs. *(Ref. 2, p. 225)*

Practice Test Questions 2

DIRECTIONS: Each of the numbered items or incomplete statements in this chapter is followed by answers or completions of the statement. Select the **ONE** lettered answer or completion that is **BEST** in each case.

AP   **151.** A maximum amount of exhalation after maximum inhalation is
   A. compensatory air
   B. residual air
   C. tidal volume
   D. vital capacity

M   **152.** Beginning anterolaterally on the arm and moving lateral to medial, the meridians are
   A. ST, LI, TW
   B. LIV, SP, KI
   C. HC, HT, LU
   D. SI, CO, SJ

M   **153.** Temperature range for hot immersion baths is **BEST** at
- **A.** 85°F–95°F
- **B.** 100°F–110°F
- **C.** 125°F–150°F
- **D.** 130°F–140°F

M   **154.** According to Beard, in superficial stroking, the direction is
- **A.** feet to head
- **B.** lateral
- **C.** of no consequence
- **D.** head to feet

P   **155.** To treat the seventh cranial palsy (Bell's palsy), brisk friction kneading should be done
- **A.** from the mandible to hairline vertically
- **B.** from the hairline to mandible
- **C.** transversely with both hands
- **D.** not at all

AP   **156.** Which of the following is **TRUE** about terminal ganglia?
- **A.** They are also know as collateral ganglia
- **B.** These ganglia receive sympathetic preganglionic fibers
- **C.** These ganglia lie close to the vertebral column and the large abdominal arteries
- **D.** These ganglia are located at the end of an autonomic motor pathway

M   **157.** In addition to massage, which is most helpful in increasing lymph flow?
- **A.** Exercise
- **B.** Heat
- **C.** Immobilization
- **D.** Passive movement

M   **158.** The therapeutic benefit of friction is
- **A.** local hyperemia
- **B.** lymphatic drainage
- **C.** tonification
- **D.** none of the above

AP **159.** In which directions do Yin meridians flow?
- **A.** Superior to inferior
- **B.** Inferior to superior
- **C.** Lateral to medial
- **D.** Medial to lateral

AP **160.** Which meridians are innervated when massaging the medial thigh?
- **A.** KI, LIV, SP
- **B.** GB, ST, SP
- **C.** LIV, ST, KI
- **D.** GB, LIV, KI

P **161.** According to Cyriax, which stroke is **BEST** for tenosynovitis?
- **A.** Effleurage
- **B.** Transverse friction
- **C.** Percussion
- **D.** Vibration

P **162.** The **BEST** massage to use on a chronic sprain is
- **A.** Effleurage
- **B.** Pick-up
- **C.** Transverse friction
- **D.** Vibration

AP **163.** Which meridian has a point on the radial side of the finger?
- **A.** Small intestine
- **B.** Triple warmer
- **C.** Heart
- **D.** Pericardium

AP **164.** The vascular system is controlled by which meridian?
- **A.** Heart
- **B.** Triple warmer
- **C.** Pericardium
- **D.** Conception vessel

AP **165.** Which meridian is involved with a system but does not have a corresponding organ?
- **A.** Spleen
- **B.** Heart

C. Liver
D. Triple heater

P   166. The stomach meridian is located between which muscles?
A. Rectus femoris and vastus medialis
B. Rectus femoris and semitendinosus
C. Rectus femoris and vastus lateralis
D. Semitendinosus and semimembranosus

M   167. On the basis of current information, the psychogenic effects of massage are **MOST LIKELY** due to
A. histamine releases
B. endorphin releases
C. local lactic acid accumulation
D. generalized vasoconstriction

P   168. Muscular dystrophy is characterized by degeneration and wasting of
A. muscle tissue
B. nervous tissue
C. epithelial tissue
D. all of the above

M   169. Which meridian is lateral to the midsagittal line of the posterior cervical vertebrae?
A. Governing vessel
B. Triple warmer
C. Stomach
D. Bladder

AP   170. Which of the following is **NOT TRUE** regarding the lumbar vertebrae?
A. They are the largest and strongest vertebrae
B. Their superior articular processes are directed superiorly instead of medially
C. Their inferior articular processes are directed laterally instead of inferiorly
D. Their spinous processes are shaped quadrilaterally

AP   **171.** Which of the following moves an extremity away from the midline?
- **A.** Adductor
- **B.** Abductor
- **C.** Flexor
- **D.** Rotator

B/E   **172.** The NCTMB code of ethics is designed to
- **A.** promote respect for the dignity of persons
- **B.** promote integrity in relationships
- **C.** promote responsible caring for clients
- **D.** all of the above

AP   **173.** Which type of joints are found in the vertebrae?
- **A.** Ball and socket
- **B.** Gliding
- **C.** Condyloid
- **D.** None of the above

AP   **174.** Thyroid hormones regulate
- **A.** the use of oxygen
- **B.** the basal metabolic rate
- **C.** the cellular metabolism
- **D.** growth and development

AP   **175.** Which is a band of strong, fibrous tissue that connects the articular ends of bones and binds them together?
- **A.** Membrane
- **B.** Fascia
- **C.** Cancellous tissue
- **D.** Ligament

P   **176.** Massage is helpful under medical supervision for which inflammatory disease?
- **A.** Rheumatoid arthritis
- **B.** Lupus
- **C.** Ankylosing spondylitis
- **D.** All of the above

AP   **177.** The carpal bones are located in the
- **A.** wrist
- **B.** foot
- **C.** ear
- **D.** sacrum

AP   **178.** The blood type that is termed the "universal recipient" is
- **A.** O
- **B.** A
- **C.** B
- **D.** AB

AP   **179.** The kidneys are located
- **A.** in the GI tract
- **B.** below 5th lumbar vertebrae
- **C.** opposite 12th thoracic vertebrae
- **D.** above the liver

P   **180.** Massage is **USUALLY** indicated for which affliction?
- **A.** Acute phlebitis
- **B.** Nausea
- **C.** Jaundice
- **D.** Sprain

M   **181.** The main purpose of deep transverse friction is to
- **A.** separate muscle fibers
- **B.** lengthen muscle fibers
- **C.** shorten muscle fibers
- **D.** minimize pain

M   **182.** *Bindegewebsmassage* is
- **A.** connective tissue massage
- **B.** reflex zone massage
- **C.** German connective tissue massage
- **D.** all of the above

M   **183.** Which stroke **MOST OFTEN** begins and ends a massage?
- **A.** Effleurage
- **B.** Petrissage
- **C.** Friction
- **D.** Vibration

AP **184.** Which of the following points is located on the nail of the first toe?
   A. ST45
   B. KI1
   C. LIV1
   D. None of the above

M **185.** What is the **BEST** massage technique to lift muscles off the bone?
   A. Effleurage
   B. Petrissage
   C. Vibration
   D. Tapotement

M **186.** What is the first **PRIMARY** consideration before beginning massage treatment?
   A. Make sure client is comfortable
   B. Make sure no jewelry is being worn
   C. Wash hands thoroughly
   D. Determine if contraindications are present

M **187.** How should you vary massage treatment with the age of the patient?
   A. Progressively with increased age
   B. Shorter with increased age
   C. Shorter for very old and very young
   D. The same for any age

M **188.** According to Hoffa,
   A. massage should last 15 minutes or less
   B. all manipulations should be gentle
   C. no point should be treated too long
   D. all of the above

M **189.** According to McMillan, what type of tapotement is done with a cupped hand?
   A. Hacking
   B. Clapping
   C. Tapping
   D. Beating

M   **190.** According to Cyriax, the **MOST** potent form of massage is
- **A.** effleurage
- **B.** petrissage
- **C.** deep traverse friction
- **D.** *shiatsu*

B/E   **191.** When opening a massage business, helpful resources include
- **A.** Chamber of Commerce
- **B.** accountant
- **C.** Small Business Administration
- **D.** all of the above

M   **192.** Which massage technique gives the **BEST** information about connective tissue structure in ligaments, tendons, and joints?
- **A.** Effleurage
- **B.** Friction
- **C.** Vibration
- **D.** Tapotement

M   **193.** Which stroke is **BEST** for breaking down adhesions?
- **A.** Effleurage
- **B.** Petrissage
- **C.** Friction
- **D.** Vibration

M   **194.** Strokes that knead are called
- **A.** effleurage
- **B.** petrissage
- **C.** friction
- **D.** vibration

P   **195.** A term that means an abnormally low level of WBCs is
- **A.** leukopenia
- **B.** leukocytopenia
- **C.** leukocytosis
- **D.** leukophoma

AP   **196.** The digestive organs drain into the
- **A.** liver (hepatic portal vein)
- **B.** aorta
- **C.** vena cava
- **D.** pulmonary artery

M   **197.** What is the **BEST** stroke for massaging the intercostals?
- **A.** Compression
- **B.** Tapotement
- **C.** Vibration
- **D.** Petrissage

AP   **198.** What is the body's normal posture called?
- **A.** Tonus
- **B.** Tetanic
- **C.** Isotonic
- **D.** Isometric

P   **199.** Tight hamstrings contribute to back pain due to
- **A.** limited lumbar movement
- **B.** ischial origin
- **C.** limited hip flexion
- **D.** all of the above

P   **200.** Carpal tunnel syndrome affects the
- **A.** volar aspect of the wrist
- **B.** dorsal wrist
- **C.** anterior forearm
- **D.** forearm extensors

AP   **201.** Myelinated axon supported by neuroglia cells are
- **A.** white matter
- **B.** gray matter
- **C.** nucleus
- **D.** ganglia

AP   **202.** Which is **NOT** connective tissue?
- **A.** Squamous epithelium
- **B.** Adipose
- **C.** Hyaline cartilage
- **D.** Tendon

P   **203.** When there is damage to the ulnar nerve with the inability to flex the fingers strongly, which condition would be present?
   - **A.** Flaccidity
   - **B.** Spasticity
   - **C.** Spasm
   - **D.** All of the above

P   **204.** Cutting the median nerve results in the inability to
   - **A.** flex the thumb
   - **B.** extend the wrist
   - **C.** extend the elbow
   - **D.** supinate the arm

P   **205.** Which is an example of a fungus infection?
   - **A.** Athlete's foot
   - **B.** Furuncle
   - **C.** Typhoid
   - **D.** Dysentery

P   **206.** Fusiform swelling in the fingers and joint calcification of the hand are seen in
   - **A.** gout
   - **B.** arthritis
   - **C.** polio
   - **D.** rheumatoid arthritis

M   **207.** How should pressure be administered during effleurage?
   - **A.** Evenly
   - **B.** Heavy decreasing to light
   - **C.** Intermittent
   - **D.** Light to heavy

M   **208.** Biofeedback is useful in
   - **A.** relieving pain through autogenic training
   - **B.** controlling involuntary processes
   - **C.** a therapeutic program
   - **D.** all of the above

AP   **209.** The **MOST** numerous formed element is
      A. thrombocytes
      B. leukocytes
      C. erythrocytes
      D. monocytes

M   **210.** Which should **NOT** be claimed as a result of massage therapy?
      A. Prevent edema
      B. Increased arterial flow
      C. Increased lymph flow
      D. Weight reduction

M   **211.** Guided imagery and meditation techniques
      A. remove blocks and stimulate healing
      B. are used for preventative treatment
      C. subliminally reinforce the mind
      D. all of the above

M   **212.** Massage can relieve pain without the use of
      A. imagery
      B. stimulation
      C. drugs, alcohol, or narcotics
      D. endorphins

M   **213.** Yoga is a form of mediation for
      A. good appetite
      B. muscle balance and relaxation
      C. dancing
      D. religion

P   **214.** Loss of function of the wrist and outer fingers is due to an injury to the
      A. brachial plexus
      B. radial nerve
      C. median nerve
      D. ulnar nerve

B/E **215.** If a massage therapist is found guilty of violation of the Massage Practice Act or Rules of Conduct, which action should be taken?
- **A.** Warning only
- **B.** Suspension of license
- **C.** Revocation of license
- **D.** All of the above

M **216.** The relaxing action of a muscle is obtained immediately by the application of
- **A.** cold
- **B.** heat
- **C.** neutral
- **D.** none of the above

M **217.** In which massage technique should the fingers move tissue under the skin but not the skin itself?
- **A.** Tapotement
- **B.** Effleurage
- **C.** Vibration
- **D.** Friction

M **218.** Deep friction massage works **BEST** if it is applied
- **A.** directly over a problem area
- **B.** proximal to a problem area
- **C.** distal to a problem area
- **D.** around the problem area

M **219.** For which type of tissue is vibration the **MOST** unsuitable?
- **A.** Major nerve course
- **B.** Reduce muscle spasm
- **C.** Bony prominences
- **D.** Skeletal muscle

M **220.** Hot compresses used immediately after injury do **NOT**
- **A.** increase blood flow
- **B.** reduce muscle spasm
- **C.** reduce swelling
- **D.** relieve pain

AP   **221.** Which meridians transverse the abdomen?
- **A.** BL, LU, TW
- **B.** HT, HC, LU
- **C.** GB, SI, CO
- **D.** KI, SP, ST

M   **222.** Which is the first step in beginning massage treatment?
- **A.** Apply lubricant
- **B.** Effleurage
- **C.** Determine contraindications
- **D.** Diagnose the patient

AP   **223.** The slippery substance that lines joint capsules is
- **A.** serous membrane
- **B.** synovial fluid
- **C.** mucus membrane
- **D.** epithelium

M   **224.** When giving CPR to a 6-year-old child, you use the
- **A.** heel of one hand
- **B.** heel of two hands
- **C.** fingers of one hand
- **D.** fingers of two hands

AP   **225.** The lymphatic system plays an important role in the production of WBC. The process is called
- **A.** osmosis
- **B.** diapedesis
- **C.** hemopoiesis
- **D.** chemical composition

AP   **226.** Although the biceps brachii is the most visible flexor, another primary muscle is
- **A.** brachialis
- **B.** pronator quadratus
- **C.** anconeus
- **D.** triceps brachii

P   **227.** A survivor of abuse can benefit from massage by
- **A.** feeling a sense of safeness
- **B.** releasing or letting go some of the abuse

         C. retrieving memory

         D. all of the above

AP   **228.** Where is the medial malleolus?

         A. Calcaneus

         B. Talus

         C. Fibula

         D. Tibia

AP   **229.** The left coronary artery arises from the

         A. ascending aorta

         B. descending aorta

         C. left atrium

         D. left ventricle

AP   **230.** Which part of a neuron carries impulses toward the cell body?

         A. Dendrite

         B. Axon

         C. Motor unit

         D. All of the above

AP   **231.** The capitulum of the humerus articulates with the

         A. radial tuberosity

         B. head of the radius

         C. olecranon of the ulna

         D. coracoid

P   **232.** Sciatic nerve injury may have symptoms of

         A. a herniated disc

         B. a dislocated hip

         C. osteoarthritis of the lumbosacral spine

         D. all of the above

M   **233.** First aid for acute soft tissue injuries involve RICE, which means

         A. ice

         B. rest and elevation

         C. compression

         D. all of the above

M   **234.** Massage treatment of chest should never be done over the
- **A.** ribs
- **B.** heart
- **C.** female nipples
- **D.** all of the above

M   **235.** Which aims **MOST** specifically to passively stretch muscle?
- **A.** Effleurage
- **B.** Friction
- **C.** Petrissage
- **D.** Tapotement

M   **236.** Massage benefits lymph flow **BEST** when strokes are
- **A.** away from heart
- **B.** toward heart
- **C.** heavy in both directions
- **D.** in certain local areas

M   **237.** For which condition is abdominal massage **MOST** beneficial?
- **A.** Pregnancy
- **B.** Appendicitis
- **C.** Constipation
- **D.** Enteritis

AP   **238.** The superior mesenteric artery supplies the
- **A.** liver and pancreas
- **B.** spleen
- **C.** small intestine, pancreas, and colon
- **D.** colon only

AP   **239.** The median nerve is part of
- **A.** the sacralplexus
- **B.** sciatic nerve
- **C.** brachial plexus
- **D.** lumbar plexus

M   **240.** In which area is massage **MOST OFTEN** used for spinal
        cord injury at T12?
        A. Chest
        B. Neck
        C. Legs
        D. Trunk

AP   **241.** The blood is filtered chemically by the
        A. kidney
        B. adrenal
        C. liver
        D. spleen

P   **242.** Shinsplint syndrome affects the
        A. lateral malleplus
        B. periosterum around the tibia
        C. fibula
        D. all of the above

AP   **243.** Where are the first and last points on the BL meridian?
        A. Head and fingers
        B. Toes and fingers
        C. Head and foot
        D. Wrist and finger

AP   **244.** Someone with a medical history of diabetes is sweat-
        ing and talking incoherently. Which liquid should you
        encourage?
        A. Water
        B. Milk
        C. Orange juice
        D. Bicarbonate of soda

P   **245.** Our emotions can lead to disease with the use of
        A. food
        B. nicotine
        C. alcohol and drugs
        D. all of the above

AP   **246.** The thoracic duct drains the
- **A.** entire body below the ribs
- **B.** head, neck, chest, left limbs
- **C.** largest lymph drainage of the body
- **D.** all of the above

AP   **247.** Which muscle is innervated by the axillary nerve?
- **A.** Deltoid
- **B.** Brachial
- **C.** Pectoralis major
- **D.** None of the above

AP   **248.** What do the following muscles have in common: SCM, biceps, brachii, hamstrings?
- **A.** Flexors
- **B.** Adductors
- **C.** Extensors
- **D.** Abductors

AP   **249.** The pancreas secretes
- **A.** insulin
- **B.** polypeptides
- **C.** glucagon
- **D.** all of the above

M   **250.** In stroking the client's anterior neck, the massage therapist has
- **A.** thumbs adducted and strokes up
- **B.** alternate hands transverse
- **C.** thumbs abducted and strokes up
- **D.** hands transverse with thumbs around esophagus

M   **251.** Which is **BEST** to prevent adhesions in muscle tissue?
- **A.** Friction and effleurage
- **B.** Friction and petrissage
- **C.** Friction and tapotement
- **D.** Friction only

M   **252.** Petrissage beginning just distal to the medial condyle and moving proximal to the gluteal fold affects which muscles?
  A. Anterior adductors
  B. Medial hamstrings
  C. Quadriceps
  D. Deltoids

AP   **253.** Lactic acid in a muscle rises in direct relation to
  A. the decrease in O_2
  B. the increase in O_2
  C. muscle sweating
  D. none of the above

M   **254.** In tapping a large area of the body, which massage maneuver is used?
  A. Percussion
  B. Friction
  C. Effleurage
  D. Petrissage

M   **255.** When applying palmar kneading to calf muscles, with the client in supine position, place a towel
  A. under the sacrum
  B. under the lower back
  C. under the knees
  D. under the ankles

M   **256.** Which condition is **ALWAYS** a contraindication for massage?
  A. Muscle spasm
  B. Phlebitis
  C. Rheumatoid arthritis
  D. Edema

AP   **257.** Which muscle bends the hand toward the wrist?
  A. Extensor carpi radialis brevis
  B. Extensor carpi radialis longus
  C. Flexor carpi radialis
  D. Flexor hallux

AP   **258.** Which is the **MOST** highly vascularized muscle tissue?
- **A.** Skeletal
- **B.** Involuntary
- **C.** Smooth
- **D.** Sphincter

P   **259.** The traumatic injury of a sprain to ligaments or a strain to a muscle tendon is a contraindication for
- **A.** avoiding area of inflammation
- **B.** evaluation by physician
- **C.** working above or below injury
- **D.** avoiding affected area

M   **260.** In massaging the anconeus, the massage practitioner is working in the area of the
- **A.** upper extremity
- **B.** lower extremity
- **C.** abdominal wall
- **D.** none of the above

AP   **261.** Which muscles are affected in a back spasm?
- **A.** Erector spinae
- **B.** Gluteus maximus and medial gluteus
- **C.** Latissimus dorsi
- **D.** Quadratus lumborum

M   **262.** For insomnia, which is **BEST**?
- **A.** Heavy effleurage
- **B.** Light effleurage
- **C.** Tapotement
- **D.** Pick-up

M   **263.** The main purpose of deep transverse friction is to
- **A.** separate muscle fibers
- **B.** lengthen muscle
- **C.** shorten muscle fibers
- **D.** minimize pain

M   **264.** Which is characteristic of a pressure stroke?
- **A.** Is of no consequence
- **B.** Follows venous flow
- **C.** Follows arterial flow
- **D.** Follows gravity

AP **265.** Adult body temperature is higher than normal at
  A. 37°C
  B. 98°F
  C. 98.6°F
  D. 39°C

M **266.** A client complains of and requests massage for severe low back pain. Which condition produces this pain and is a contraindication for massage?
  A. Phlebitis
  B. Postural deviation
  C. Herniated disc
  D. Torticollis

AP **267.** The triple warmer controls
  A. assimilation, digestion, elimination
  B. assimilation, digestion, skin temperature regulation
  C. digestion, elimination, skin temperature regulation
  D. elimination, digestion, nervous system

AP **268.** Which muscle abducts the scapula?
  A. Serratus anterior/pectoralis minor
  B. Rhomboids
  C. Latissimus dorsi
  D. Trapezius

AP **269.** Which is (are) not a part of the central nervous system (CNS)?
  A. Cranial nerves
  B. Cerebellum
  C. White tracts
  D. Medulla oblongata

AP **270.** Which divides the thorax from the abdomen?
  A. Diaphragm
  B. Ribs
  C. Lungs
  D. None of the above

P   **271.** Somatic pain arises from stimulation of
       A. organ receptors
       B. noxious material
       C. receptors of the skin, muscles, or joints
       D. referred areas

M   **272.** To massage the hand, use
       A. effleurage and petrissage
       B. compression
       C. ROM and circular friction
       D. all of the above

AP   **273.** The external iliac artery supplies blood to
       A. the lower limbs
       B. all parts of the trunk
       C. the neck and back
       D. the pelvic organs

M   **274.** To massage the elderly, which stroke would you use?
       A. Tapotement
       B. Gentle effleurage and petrissage
       C. Deep pressure
       D. Friction over pressure area

AP   **275.** What plantarflexes and everts the foot?
       A. Tibialis anterior
       B. Gastrocnemius
       C. Plantaris
       D. Peroneus longus

P   **276.** In pregnancy a contraindication for prenatal massage is
       A. varicose veins
       B. toxemia
       C. dizziness
       D. all of the above

AP   **277.** Manipulation of the sacral area **MOST** directly affects energy in which meridian?
       A. BL
       B. GNB

C. KI
D. ST

AP   **278.** The normal resting pulse rate range is
     A. 70–80 beats per minute
     B. 80–90 beats per minute
     C. 120–130 beats per minute
     D. all of the above

AP   **279.** Which muscle extends the femur?
     A. Soleus
     B. Gluteus minimus
     C. Gluteus maximus
     D. Peroneus

AP   **280.** What is the normal systolic pressure?
     A. 80 mm/Hg
     B. 90 mm/Hg
     C. 120 mm/Hg
     D. 140 mm/Hg

M   **281.** When palpating the midline of the back, what is being touched?
     A. Transverse process
     B. Vertebral body
     C. Spinous process
     D. Articular joint

M   **282.** Mild stimulation of the vagus nerve results in
     A. irregular heartbeat
     B. no change
     C. increased heartbeat
     D. decreased heartbeat

AP   **283.** Which muscle inserts into the iliotibial band?
     A. Gluteus maximus
     B. Quadratus femoris
     C. Gluteus medias
     D. Tensor fascia latae

P   **284.** The following deviations that suggest the need for evaluation and referral for cardiovascular clients are
   A. pulse over 90 or under 60
   B. red, warm, or hard veins
   C. pain and tenderness of extremities
   D. all of the above

AP   **285.** Which of the following is (are) **NOT** found in the dermis?
   A. Blood vessels
   B. Nerve endings
   C. Striated muscle
   D. Hair roots

AP   **286.** The diaphragm contracts on
   A. inspiration
   B. expiration
   C. both
   D. neither

M   **287.** Contraindications for hydrotherapy do **NOT** include which of the following?
   A. Kidney infection
   B. Cold
   C. High or low blood pressure
   D. Skin infection

M   **288.** Massage therapy is used in pain management for
   A. cardiac and terminal cancer patients
   B. posttrauma patients
   C. postsurgical patients
   D. all of the above

M   **289.** The use of cold to depress the activity of pain receptors in the treatment of myofascial pain
   A. maintains skin temperature of 13.6°C
   B. increases nerve conduction velocity
   C. permits passive stretching and exercise
   D. decreases the general activity of patient

AP **290.** Coronary sinus receives almost all venous blood from the
    A. brain
    B. brachiocephalic veins
    C. inferior vena cava
    D. myocardium

M **291.** The primary physiological effect of massage therapy includes all **EXCEPT**
    A. delivery of oxygen to cells
    B. clearance of metabolic waste and by-product of tissue damage
    C. increased blood and lymph circulation
    D. increased interstitial fluid and hydrostatic pressure

M **292.** Vodder's manual lymph drainage (MLD) was developed for the specific purpose of
    A. promoting lymph flow from tissue
    B. eliminating the pneumatic cuff
    C. decreasing urine output
    D. increasing erythrocyte count

P **293.** Flaccid paralysis can be benefited by the
    A. decrease in metabolic heat production
    B. increase in heart rate and blood pressure
    C. deep stroking and kneading massage
    D. relaxation of muscle tissue

AP **294.** Histamines
    A. act as chemotactic agents
    B. form membrane attach complex
    C. increase permeability of blood capillaries
    D. cause cytolysis of white blood cells

P **295.** Myofascial pain syndrome is also known as
    A. myofascitis
    B. fibromyositis
    C. myofascitis trigger points
    D. all of the above

AP **296.** The PQRST wave is
A. the triple heater meridian
B. conduction through the heart
C. a nerve impulse
D. none of the above

AP **297.** People who have been inactive for extended periods and engage in sporadic physical exercise suffer from
A. DMS (delayed muscle soreness)
B. muscle spasm with tissue ischemia
C. damage to muscle fiber
D. all of the above

P **298.** Fibrosis, the formation of abnormal collagenous connective tissue, is **BEST** treated by
A. deep friction massage
B. passive movements
C. kneading
D. all of the above

P **299.** Pain sensations are modified by the release of neurochemicals from the CNS, including
A. adrenalin
B. endorphins and enkephlins
C. thyroxin
D. prostaglandins

M **300.** The analgesic effect of ice massage is to
A. block pain impulse conduction
B. reroute pain
C. decrease ROM
D. eliminate pain

Practice Test Questions 2

Answers and Discussion

151. (D) The maximum air volume that can be expelled is the vital capacity of the lungs. The intercostal muscles and abdominal muscle contract as the diaphragm moves up. *(Ref. 2, p. 227)*

152. (A) The stomach, large intestine, and triple warmer are meridians that travel from the lateral arm to the median part of the anterior body. *(Ref. 5, pp. 137–139)*

153. (B) The temperature best for nerves, insomnia, and aching muscles is 100°F–110°F. This induces relaxation and relieves nervous tension. *(Ref. 2, p. 473)*

154. (A) To promote good circulation, the effleurage stroke should begin from the lower extremity and move up toward the head. *(Ref. 5, p. 69)*

155. (A) In Bell's palsy, the paralyzed side of the mouth area is stretched, and massage should be on both sides from the mandible to the hairline in a kneading stroke. *(Ref. 2, p. 195; Ref. 5, p. 106)*

156. (D) Terminal ganglia are located at the end of an autonomic motor pathway. *(Ref. 8, p. 505)*

157. (A) Exercise stimulates lymph flow due to muscle contracting on the lymph vessels, forcing the movement of the lymph. *(Ref. 2, p. 544)*

158. (A) A form of friction called compression increases circulation and lasting hyperemia in the tissue. The pumping action brings blood to deep muscles for long periods. *(Ref. 2, p. 320)*

159. (B) The flow of energy for the Yin meridians is from the inferior part of the body to the superior. *(Ref. 2, p. 564)*

160. (A) The kidney, liver, and spleen are the meridians that pass through the medial thigh area. *(Ref. 2, p. 566)*

161. (B) Deep transverse friction should be used to break up scar tissue from overuse in tenosynovitis. *(Ref. 5, p. 264)*

162. (C) Transverse friction massage is the best method to keep adhesions and scar tissue from forming, as well as to promote healing in a sprain. *(Ref. 2, p. 521)*

163. (C) The heart meridian has a point on the little finger, and energy flows from the chest to the inside of the arm. *(Ref. 2, p. 566; Ref. 5, p. 139)*

164. (A) The heart meridian follows the flow of blood from the chest to the arm to the end of the little finger. *(Ref. 5, p. 139)*

165. (D) The triple heater (warmer) is the meridian that stands for fire and has no corresponding organ along the energy path from the ring finger to the side of the head. *(Ref. 2, p. 566)*

166. (C) The rectus femoris is separated from the vastus lateralis muscle by the stomach meridian. *(Ref. 2, p. 566)*

167. (B) The morphinelike substance, endorphin, is released by the limbic system at the base of the brain stem and produces reduction in pain and a feeling of well-being. *(Ref. 5, p. 45)*

168. (A) The muscle tissue degenerates during muscular dystrophy as a result of muscle atrophy. *(Ref. 2, p. 123)*

169. **(D)** The bladder meridian is lateral to the midsagittal line of the posterior cervical vertebrae. *(Ref. 2, p. 566)*

170. **(B)** The lumbar vertebrae articulate directly medially instead of superiorly. *(Ref. 8, p. 190)*

171. **(B)** The abductor muscles move an appendage away from the body. *(Ref. 2, pp. 43, 138)*

172. **(D)** All massage therapists should follow the code of ethics concerning respect, integrity, and caring after obtaining national certification. *(Ref. 11, p. 38)*

173. **(B)** The vertebrae are slightly movable joints that are classified as gliding. *(Ref. 3, p. 33)*

174. **(D)** The hormone that regulates growth and development is thyroxine. *(Ref. 8, p. 535)*

175. **(D)** A ligament is the strong fibrous connective tissue that articulates bone to bone. *(Ref. 2, p. 98)*

176. **(D)** Many diseases cause inflammation of tissue and massage is beneficial. They include Lupus, spondylitis, and arthritis. *(Ref. 11, pp. 398–399)*

177. **(A)** The eight bones that make up the wrist are called carpals. *(Ref. 3, p. 7)*

178. **(D)** A person who is able to receive blood from any other blood type is AB and is the universal recipient. *(Ref. 8, p. 585)*

179. **(C)** The kidneys are located in the abdominal cavity just posterior to the floating ribs and adjacent to T-12. *(Ref. 3, p. 108)*

180. **(D)** An appropriate treatment for a sprain is massage therapy. *(Ref. 2, pp. 100–101)*

181. **(A)** To separate muscle fibers from an injury or scar, transverse friction is the recommended therapy. *(Ref. 2, p. 318)*

182. **(D)** The technique called *Bindegewebsmassage* manipulates reflex zones and connective tissue. *(Ref. 5, pp. 219–254)*

183. (A) The stroke that usually begins and ends a massage is effleurage. *(Ref. 2, p. 312)*

184. (C) The liver (LIV) meridian is located on the big toe. *(Ref. 2, p. 566)*

185. (B) Petrissage is the best stroke to lift the muscle off the bones. *(Ref. 2, p. 316)*

186. (D) Massage should not begin if any contraindication is present. *(Ref. 2, p. 487)*

187. (C) Treatment to the old and young should be shortened. They are more fragile and cannot endure a lengthy session. *(Ref. 2, p. 77)*

188. (D) Hoffa designed a massage technique that is short, gentle, and quick to each area. *(Ref. 5, p. 268)*

189. (B) The cupped hand technique claps the skin and is characteristic of McMillan. *(Ref. 5, p. 279)*

190. (C) The massage technique that Cyriax feels is effective is deep traverse friction. *(Ref. 5, p. 261)*

191. (D) Many consultants are available when opening a business including an attorney, the SBA, an accountant, and Chambers of Commerce. *(Ref. 11, p. 150)*

192. (B) Friction allows the fingers to feel the tissues below due to the deeper pressure applied. *(Ref. 2, p. 319)*

193. (C) To loosen adhesion tissue, cross-fiber friction is the best stroke to mobilize the area. *(Ref. 2, p. 318)*

194. (B) In the petrissage stroke, the tissue is lifted up off the bone in a kneading technique. *(Ref. 2, p. 315)*

195. (A) If the level of WBCs becomes lower than normal, the result is leukopenia. *(Ref. 8, p. 577)*

196. (A) Blood returns to the heart through the hepatic portal system when digestion is completed. *(Ref. 3, p. 74)*

197. **(A)** Compression is an excellent massage for the intercostal muscles of the ribs. The pumping action provides improvement of breathing. *(Ref. 2, p. 533)*

198. **(A)** Tonus is good muscle tone necessary for body posture. *(Ref. 8, p. 249)*

199. **(D)** Back pain and tight hamstrings are the result of limited hip and lumbar movement. *(Ref. 3, p. 54)*

200. **(A)** The volar area of the wrist is affected in carpal tunnel syndrome. *(Ref. 8, p. 312)*

201. **(A)** The white matter is collectively the axons that are supported by the neuroglia cells. *(Ref. 3, pp. 11, 138)*

202. **(A)** Squamous epithelium is one of the epithelial tissue types, not a connective tissue. *(Ref. 2, pp. 58–59)*

203. **(A)** Lack of muscle movement due to nerve damage is called flaccidity. *(Ref. 2, p. 199)*

204. **(A)** The median nerve in the arm is responsible for motion and sensation of the thumb, index, and middle finger. If it is cut, the thumb does not have the ability to flex. *(Ref. 2, pp. 199, 209)*

205. **(A)** Athlete's foot is a fungus infection that attacks the foot and toes. *(Ref. 8, p. 141)*

206. **(D)** Rheumatoid arthritis is a chronic inflammatory disease of the joint with cartilage erosion and eventual immobilization. *(Ref. 2, p. 101)*

207. **(D)** The pressure during effleurage should initially be lighter than at the end of the stroke or manipulation. *(Ref. 2, p. 347)*

208. **(D)** Biofeedback has many therapeutic uses, including pain relief through autogenic training and aid in controlling involuntary processes. *(Ref. 5, p. 48)*

209. **(C)** There are approximately 5×10^6 mm^3 erythrocytes and 10,000 mm^3 WBCs in the blood. *(Ref. 8, p. 570)*

210. **(D)** Massage therapy helps to tone muscles and improve circulation, but does not alone guarantee weight loss. *(Ref. 2, p. 253)*

211. **(D)** Imagery and meditation are techniques used to remove blocks, stimulate healing, and subliminally reinforce the mind. *(Ref. 5, p. 50)*

212. **(C)** Endorphins can relieve pain without the use of drugs, alcohol, or narcotics. *(Ref. 5, p. 45)*

213. **(B)** When yoga is practiced, the result can be muscle balance and relaxation. *(Ref. 2, p. 603)*

214. **(D)** The ulnar nerve travels through the arms, wrists, and fingers. Any injury to this area prevents the function of the wrist or outer fingers. *(Ref. 2, p. 209)*

215. **(D)** Violating massage Rules of Conduct can result in a warning, suspension, or revocation of license. *(Ref. 2, p. 23)*

216. **(B)** Heat to the muscle area stimulates the muscle to relax. *(Ref. 2, p. 460)*

217. **(D)** Friction is the massage stroke that moves the fascia and tissue under the skin without moving the skin itself. *(Ref. 2, p. 318)*

218. **(D)** The best massage technique to use around a problem area is deep friction, due to aiding blood flow and absorption of the fluid. *(Ref. 2, p. 319)*

219. **(C)** Bony prominences are too sensitive for vibration massage. *(Ref. 2, p. 324)*

220. **(C)** Hot compresses do not reduce swelling from an injured area; they vasodilate, raising body temperature in an attempt to dissipate the heat. *(Ref. 2, pp. 460–464)*

221. **(D)** The kidney, spleen, and stomach are the meridians that transverse the abdomen. *(Ref. 2, p. 566)*

222. (C) All contraindications should be determined before giving a massage treatment. *(Ref. 2, p. 253)*

223. (B) The synovial fluid is responsible for the lubrication at the joints capsule. *(Ref. 2, p. 97)*

224. (A) Only the heel of one hand should be used when administering CPR to a child of 6 years. *(Ref. 1)*

225. (C) Hemopoiesis is the process of blood cell production in the bone marrow. *(Ref. 2, p. 36)*

226. (A) The brachialis is an important flexor of the arm, along with the biceps brachii. *(Ref. 3, p. 49)*

227. (D) Survivors of abuse benefit from the touch of massage because it triggers many feelings and emotions. *(Ref. 10, pp. 84–85)*

228. (D) The medial malleolus is found on the medial side of the tibia in the leg. *(Ref. 2, p. 95)*

229. (A) The ascending aorta gives rise to many arteries, including the left coronary artery of the heart. *(Ref. 2, p. 166)*

230. (A) The dendrite is the structure on the neuron that carries impulses toward the cell body. *(Ref. 2, p. 190)*

231. (B) The head of the radius articulates with the humerus at the capitulum. *(Ref. 8, p. 203)*

232. (D) Lumbar pain, a dislocated hip, and a herniated disc are all symptomatic of injury to the sciatic nerve. *(Ref. 8, p. 398)*

233. (D) RICE is an acronym for rest, ice, compression, and elevation. *(Ref. 2, p. 522)*

234. (C) In females, massage of the nipple area is omitted. *(Ref. 2, p. 412)*

235. (A) Effleurage is the massage stroke that passively moves and stretches muscles. *(Ref. 2, p. 310)*

236. (B) A benefit of massage is that, when the stroke is toward the heart, blood drains from the venous system and lymph from the lymphatic. *(Ref. 2, p. 183)*

237. (C) A benefit of abdominal massage is alleviating constipation. *(Ref. 2, p. 414)*

238. (C) The small intestine, pancreas, and colon receive blood from the superior mesenteric artery. *(Ref. 3, p. 74)*

239. (C) The brachial plexus has many nerves that go into the shoulder and arm, including the median nerve. *(Ref. 3, p. 130)*

240. (C) The lumbar plexus supplies innervation to the legs and it is best to massage the lumbar area around T12. *(Ref. 8, p. 398)*

241. (A) Blood enters the kidney via the renal artery and is filtered in the cortex and medulla by the microscopic nephron. *(Ref. 3, p. 110)*

242. (B) Inflammation of the periosteum around the tibia is one symptom of shinsplints. *(Ref. 8, p. 341)*

243. (C) The bladder meridian energy flow travels on the posterior side, starting on the head, down the back, along the leg to the toe. *(Ref. 2, p. 566)*

244. (C) Orange juice, which is high in glucose, is the liquid to give a person with hyperinsulinism. *(Ref. 8, p. 551)*

245. (D) People use chemical substances to help our feelings and in turn alter our emotions, but the use of excess food, drugs, and nicotine can lead to disease. *(Ref. 11, p. 386)*

246. (B) The lymph drainage of the head, neck, chest, and left limbs drains into the thoracic duct. *(Ref. 2, p. 56)*

247. (A) The axillary nerve is part of the brachial plexus that innervates the deltoid at the shoulder. *(Ref. 8, p. 340)*

248. (A) Muscles that reduce the angle of muscle actions are called flexors. The SCM, biceps brachii, and hamstrings are all flexors. *(Ref. 2, p. 142)*

249. **(D)** The pancreas is an endocrine gland secreting insulin to glucagon hormones, as well as functioning as a digestive organ secreting polypeptides. *(Ref. 8, p. 552)*

250. **(C)** The massage at the neck is given with the thumbs abducted with a bilateral effleurage stroke beginning at the sternal notch over the shoulders and up the neck. *(Ref. 2, p. 393)*

251. **(A)** Friction and effleurage can prevent scarring and adhesions to muscle tissue due to the action of keeping the fiber separated by either cross-fiber or longitudinal strokes. *(Ref. 2, p. 319)*

252. **(B)** Petrissage proximal to the gluteal muscles is effective on the hamstrings. *(Ref. 2, p. 420)*

253. **(A)** When the muscle goes into oxygen debt, the lactic acid builds up from the anaerobic component of cell respiration. *(Ref. 8, p. 253)*

254. **(A)** Percussion includes tapping, slapping, hacking, cupping, and beating, which benefit a large area like the back. *(Ref. 2, p. 492)*

255. **(C)** When the client is in the supine position, a towel is placed under the knees so that palmar kneading is possible. *(Ref. 2, p. 373)*

256. **(B)** Phlebitis is always a contraindication for massage. Inflammation in the veins or a possible clot is a dangerous condition. *(Ref. 2, p. 256)*

257. **(C)** The hand flexes toward the wrist with the flexor carpi radialis. *(Ref. 2, p. 257)*

258. **(A)** Skeletal muscle is rich in blood for quick movement, which requires ATP and gas exchange. *(Ref. 8, p. 257)*

259. **(B)** A physician must evaluate sprains and strains before massage treatment is applied. *(Ref. 11, p. 398)*

260. **(A)** Extending the elbow is the action of the anconeus in the upper arm, which originates on the humerus. *(Ref. 2, p. 129)*

261. **(A)** In a back spasm, kneading around the spine is important. Vibrate and hack on the erector spinae muscles. *(Ref. 2, p. 427)*

262. **(B)** Light strokes to the forehead are good for nervous headaches and insomnia; gentle gliding strokes are beneficial. *(Ref. 2, p. 312)*

263. **(A)** The transverse action of friction is applied across muscle and tendon to separate fibers, allowing greater circulation and increased mobility. *(Ref. 2, p. 318)*

264. **(D)** The slightest pressure is transmitted to deeper muscles by gravity. *(Ref. 2, p. 313)*

265. **(D)** Any body temperature above 98.6°F or 37°C is higher than normal body temperature. *(Ref. 8, p. 856)*

266. **(C)** When the fibrocartilage of the intervertebral disc is herniated, lower lumbar pain contraindicates massage in that area of the back. *(Ref. 8, p. 195)*

267. **(C)** The Yang meridian triple warmer goes from the ring finger back to the side of the head, controlling temperature, digestion, and elimination. *(Ref. 2, p. 566)*

268. **(A)** Abduction of the scapula is controlled by the pectoralis minor and serratus anterior. *(Ref. 2, p. 124)*

269. **(A)** The 12 pairs of cranial nerves are motor or sensory, and arise from the base of the brain apart from the CNS. *(Ref. 2, p. 191)*

270. **(A)** The thoracic cavity is separated from the abdominal cavity by the diaphragm muscle. *(Ref. 8, p. 18)*

271. **(C)** The cortex back to the stimulated area projects somatic pain. *(Ref. 11, p. 95)*

272. **(D)** A complete massage to the hand is effleurage, circular friction to the back of the hand, petrissage ROM, and compression to wrist and fingers. *(Ref. 2, p. 400)*

273. **(A)** The iliac branches off the dorsal aorta to supply the legs. *(Ref. 2, p. 175)*

274. **(B)** Gentle massage is beneficial to the elderly, even if they are frail. *(Ref. 2, p. 259)*

275. **(D)** The peroneus longus is responsible for the eversion of the foot and the plantar flexion. *(Ref. 2, p. 145)*

276. **(D)** Even though massage is recommended for pregnancy, many contraindications are possible and need a doctor's attention. *(Ref. 2, p. 541)*

277. **(A)** The bladder meridian is massaged to affect energy as well as for sacral pain. *(Ref. 5, p. 140)*

278. **(A)** The adult normal pulse range is 70–80 beats per minute. *(Ref. 8, p. 645)*

279. **(C)** The gluteus maximus is an extender of the hip and femur. *(Ref. 2, p. 138)*

280. **(C)** Blood pressure is measured in systolic and diastolic measurements. A normal systolic pressure is 120 mm/Hg and diastolic 80 mm/Hg. *(Ref. 8, p. 646)*

281. **(C)** The spinal process runs along the midline of the back when palpating is recommended. *(Ref. 8, p. 319)*

282. **(D)** The vagus nerve is the tenth cranial nerve, which acts as a decelerator. *(Ref. 8, p. 611)*

283. **(D)** The iliotibial band is inserted by the tensor fascia latae. *(Ref. 2, p. 138)*

284. **(D)** Any client who suffers from a cardiovascular deviation of any type needs a referral. *(Ref. 11, p. 404)*

285. **(C)** The dermis of the skin is vascular and does not contain any muscle. *(Ref. 2, p. 74)*

286. (A) The diaphragm is a smooth muscle in breathing and contracts during inspiration (moves down). *(Ref. 2, p. 227)*

287. (B) Hydrotherapy is the use of any form of water or temperature of water, cold or hot. *(Ref. 2, p. 471)*

288. (D) Massage therapy is used for posttrauma and postsurgical patients, as well as for cancer and cardiac patients. *(Ref. 9, p. 27)*

289. (C) Cold depresses pain receptors, allowing treatment by passive stretching. *(Ref. 9, p. 27)*

290. (C) The coronary sinus receives the venous blood from the inferior vena cava. *(Ref. 8, p. 660)*

291. (D) Interstitial fluid and hydrostatic pressure increases are not significant physiological effects of massage. *(Ref. 9, p. 1)*

292. (A) To shift edema fluid from tissues to blood, Vodder (in 1965), designed the MLD (manual lymph drainage.) *(Ref. 2, p. 541; Ref. 9, p. 3)*

293. (C) Increasing circulation by deep stroking and kneading aids flaccid paralysis in limbs. *(Ref. 9, p. 8)*

294. (C) Histamines are vasodilators and can therefore increase the permeability of the capillaries. *(Ref. 8, p. 693)*

295. (D) Myofascial pain includes a plethora of terms: myositis, myofascitis, and fibromyositis. *(Ref. 9, p. 13)*

296. (B) The cardiac cycle is recorded as an ECG made of the PQRST wave of one beat. The R=systole, T=diastole. *(Ref. 3, p. 67)*

297. (A) When there is muscle discomfort 24 to 48 hours after exercise, the diagnosis is DMS (delayed muscle soreness.) *(Ref. 9, p. 15)*

298. (D) Fibrosis can be mobilized by CTM, kneading, and friction. *(Ref. 9, pp. 18–19)*

299. (B) The neurochemicals, endorphines and enkephlins, relieve pain and act as an analgesia. *(Ref. 9, p. 25)*

300. (A) Ice is used to block pain before massaging an area. *(Ref. 9, p. 26)*

Practice Test Questions 3

DIRECTIONS: Each of the numbered items or incomplete statements in this chapter is followed by answers or completions of the statement. Select the **ONE** lettered answer or completion that is **BEST** in each case.

P   **301.** Massage therapy is used for pain control in
    A. labor and delivery
    B. neuritis, neuralgia
    C. whiplash
    D. all of the above

AP   **302.** Lymph is interstitial fluid consisting of
    A. water, cell debris, gases, metabolic wastes, bacteria
    B. water and gas
    C. blood, lymphocytes, bacteria
    D. water alone

M 303. Correct lymph massage begins at the
A. left thoracic duct
B. right arm
C. groin
D. right thoracic duct at the clavicle

B/E 304. Business expenses can include the cost of
A. business cards and advertising
B. professional clothes and linens
C. license, insurance, and memberships
D. all of the above

B/E 305. Client files are important for
A. record keeping for the Internal Revenue Service
B. keeping well informed of client's needs
C. documenting your "work" on clients
D. all of the above

B/E 306. Good bookkeeping for healing arts professionals can
A. eliminate tracking sheets
B. decrease bank statements
C. increase petty cash fund
D. increase legitimate tax deductions

B/E 307. If you are a self-employed massage therapist, you must file
A. no returns at all
B. only Schedule C—Profit or Loss
C. Form 1040 and Social Security Self-Employment Tax Form
D. B and C

B/E 308. Techniques to market professional skills include
A. publications and presentations
B. business cards and brochures
C. donation of services
D. all of the above

B/E   **309.** Good client records should include the
       A. intake form
       B. intake, health information, treatment and session notes
       C. client history
       D. payments received

B/E   **310.** A typical client intake form should include
       A. name and address
       B. name, address, occupation, physician, emergency number
       C. name, phone, hobbies
       D. name, marital status, children

M   **311.** Massage can be effective in all **EXCEPT** which of the following?
       A. Facilitating rehabilitation
       B. Inhibiting a psychological effect
       C. Preparing healthy muscles for strenuous activity
       D. Enhancing the healing process

M   **312.** The purpose of a lubricant when massaging is to
       A. keep the body greasy
       B. prevent blisters from forming
       C. cleanse the body for relaxation
       D. avoid uncomfortable friction between the therapist's hand and the patient's skin

B/E   **313.** A massage therapist or bodyworker can claim business deductions on Schedule C for
       A. cost of massage table, linens, and oils
       B. all vacations
       C. professional convention fees
       D. A and C

P   **314.** A systemic inflammatory disease is a chronic condition such as
       A. arthritis
       B. bronchitis
       C. asthma
       D. all of the above

M 315. Massage helps the skin to return to its normal function by
   A. slowing the metabolism
   B. removing excretory products and dead skin
   C. decreasing hair growth
   D. eliminating scar tissue from forming

AP 316. Endorphins, which act like morphine for pain relief, are released from the
   A. ANS
   B. midbrain
   C. limbic system and brain stem
   D. CNS

M 317. A unidirectional flow stroke, returning through the air, is characteristic of
   A. Cyriax
   B. Hoffa
   C. Leer
   D. Mennell

M 318. The purpose of the effleurage in massage is
   A. relaxation
   B. ROM
   C. search for spasms and spread lubricant
   D. apply pressure to the spine

M 319. The kneading motion of petrissage serves to "milk" the muscle and
   A. remove waste products
   B. assist abnormal inactivity
   C. assist venous return
   D. all of the above

P 320. The intake history of a client suffering from childhood abuse is very important because
   A. you can act as a psychotherapist
   B. it defines client boundaries and assures protection
   C. it is easy for a client to receive a massage
   D. you will be able to make a diagnosis

AP   **321.** Which major body system regulates the volume and chemical composition of blood, eliminates waste, regulates fluid and electrolyte balance, and helps regulate red blood cell count?

     A. Cardiovascular
     B. Digestive
     C. Muscular
     D. Urinary

AP   **322.** Which term means "on the opposite side of the body"?

     A. Contralateral
     B. Distal
     C. Intermediate
     D. Proximal

M   **323.** A light compressive force applied to the skin with one hand to release a dysfunction in the connective tissue is associated with

     A. myofascial releases
     B. Upledger Institute
     C. John Barnes
     D. all of the above

AP   **324.** Which muscle is **NOT** part of the rotator cuff?

     A. Supraspinatus
     B. Infraspinatus
     C. Teres major
     D. Teres minor

AP   **325.** The homeostatic responses of the body are regulated by which two systems?

     A. Digestive, urinary
     B. Reproductive, endocrine
     C. Endocrine, nervous
     D. Cardiovascular, respiratory

P   **326.** A massage therapist needs to know that the mechanism of pain includes

     A. physiological aspects
     B. social aspects
     C. psychological aspects
     D. all of the above

B/E   **327.** In opening a massage office, it is essential to investigate
      certain requirements including
      A. zoning
      B. fire inspection
      C. licensing laws
      D. all of the above

AP   **328.** The most abundant inorganic substance in humans is
      A. carbohydrate
      B. lipid
      C. oxygen
      D. water

AP   **329.** Which of the following is an acidic pH?
      A. 14
      B. 12
      C. 10
      D. 6

AP   **330.** Small, thin-walled tubes that collect lymph from intersti-
      tial fluid are called
      A. lymph capillaries
      B. sweat glands
      C. blood plasma
      D. bronchial tubes

M   **331.** Neck mobilization in a lateral flexion helps to stretch the
      cervical muscles and the
      A. trapezium
      B. deltoid
      C. occipital
      D. rhomboids

AP   **332.** The Tendino-Muscle Channels of the lung pass through
      muscles of the chest and arm that include
      A. pectorals
      B. biceps brochii
      C. diaphragm
      D. all of the above

M   **333.** The all-purpose clean up of bodily fluids is
   A. 2% bleach solution
   B. 10% bleach solution
   C. distilled water
   D. concentrated bleach

AP   **334.** In oxygen's presence, glucose is completely broken down into which two elements?
   A. Hydrogen, water
   B. Helium, sulfur
   C. Oxygen, calcium
   D. Carbon dioxide, water

AP   **335.** A class of proteins that serves to immunize the body against specific antigens is called
   A. antibodies
   B. anybodies
   C. nobodies
   D. pathogens

AP   **336.** The Governing Vessel is the confluence of all the
   A. Yin channels
   B. Yang channels
   C. Qi energy
   D. five elements

M   **337.** After the massage is complete, the therapist will
   A. escort the client to the bathroom
   B. withdraw from the client by using body language
   C. help dress the client
   D. ask the client if he did a good job

AP   **338.** Which of the following is a connective tissue cell that produces histamine?
   A. Adipocyte
   B. Fibroblast
   C. Macrophage
   D. Mast cell

AP **339.** The epidermis is composed of
   A. simple squamous epithelium
   B. simple cuboidal epithelium
   C. simple columnar epithelium
   D. stratified squamous epithelium

AP **340.** Which of the following is **TRUE** about aging of the integumentary system starting with the late forties?
   A. Collagen fibers increase
   B. Elasticity increases in elastic fibers
   C. Fibroblasts decrease in number
   D. Hair and nail growth tends to speed up

P **341.** A first-degree burn is characterized by
   A. involvement of the dermis and epidermis
   B. blisters
   C. severe pain
   D. a typical sunburn

P **342.** A second-degree burn is characterized by
   A. involvement of the entire epidermis and possibly some of the dermis
   B. no loss of skin functions
   C. damage to most hair follicles and sweat glands
   D. never scarring

M **343.** A thorough preliminary client assessment includes
   A. client history
   B. client observation
   C. client examination
   D. all of the above

AP **344.** A detailed map of the foot was developed by Ingham as *Zone Therapy* in the years preceding World War II. She then traveled across the U.S. teaching workshops on
   A. reflexology
   B. polarity
   C. Amma therapy
   D. Shiatsu

AP   **345.** What is the primary salt that makes bone matrix hard?
       A. Calcium carbonate
       B. Potassium chloride
       C. Sodium chloride
       D. None of the above

P   **346.** What is the name of the fracture of the distal end of the radius in which the distal fragment is displaced posteriorly?
       A. Stress fracture
       B. Spiral fracture
       C. Pott's fracture
       D. Colle's fracture

P   **347.** Which of the following is defined as the degeneration of cartilage allowing the bony ends to touch, and usually associated with the elderly?
       A. Osteoarthritis
       B. Osteogenic sarcoma
       C. Osteomyelitis
       D. Osteopenia

AP   **348.** Which of the following proceses forms a joint?
       A. Meatus
       B. Crest
       C. Tuberosity
       D. Condyle

P   **349.** Limitation due to the stretching of fibrous tissues is called
       A. hard end feel
       B. springy end feel
       C. soft end feel
       D. acute inflammation

AP   **350.** Which of the following are paired cranial bones?
       A. Occipital and sphenoid
       B. Temporal and parietal
       C. Frontal and ethmoid
       D. Parietal and ethmoid

AP   **351.** Which of the following is **TRUE** with regard to the humerus?
- **A.** The olecranon fossa is an anterior depression that receives the ulna's olecranon process
- **B.** The medial and lateral epicondyles are rough projections on either side of the proximal end
- **C.** The radial fossa is a posterior depression that receives the head of the radius when the forearm is flexed
- **D.** Its trochlea articulates with the ulna

AP   **352.** The prominence felt on the medial surface of the ankle is the
- **A.** fibular notch
- **B.** medial condyle
- **C.** medial malleolus
- **D.** tarsus

AP   **353.** The largest and strongest tarsal bone is the
- **A.** calcaneus
- **B.** cuboid
- **C.** lateral cuneiform
- **D.** navicular

AP   **354.** Which of the following joint classifications is described as freely movable?
- **A.** Amphiarthrosis
- **B.** Cartilaginous
- **C.** Diarthrosis
- **D.** Fibrous

AP   **355.** The joint between the trapezium carpal bone and the thumb's metacarpal is which kind of joint?
- **A.** Ball-and-socket
- **B.** Ellipsoidal
- **C.** Gliding
- **D.** Saddle

AP   **356.** Which subtype of diarthroses joint is found in the knee, elbow, and ankle?
- **A.** Ball-and-socket
- **B.** Ellipsoidal
- **C.** Gliding
- **D.** Hinge

AP   **357.** Which of the following is an intraarticular ligament of the knee?
- **A.** Anterior cruciate
- **B.** Arcuate popliteal
- **C.** Medial collateral
- **D.** Oblique popliteal

P   **358.** Which ligament is stretched or torn in about 70% of all serious knee injuries?
- **A.** Anterior cruciate
- **B.** Arculate popliteal
- **C.** Lateral collateral
- **D.** Medial collateral

P   **359.** When injured by trauma or infection, neurons of the central nervous system
- **A.** repair slowly
- **B.** don't repair
- **C.** require transplants
- **D.** self-destruct

AP   **360.** Which of the following is **TRUE** concerning the microscopic anatomy of skeletal muscle?
- **A.** A sarcolemma is the muscle fiber's cytoplasm
- **B.** The skeletal muscle fiber is a long, cylindrical cell
- **C.** The sarcoplasma is the muscle fiber's plasma membrane
- **D.** Each skeletal muscle cell has several nuclei

AP   **361.** A critical principle of holistic health is that the mind and body
- **A.** are separate from the organs
- **B.** function independently
- **C.** are seen as a single entity
- **D.** force the healing process

AP   **362.** The Ki flow through the meridians is the
- **A.** Hara breathing meditation
- **B.** blockage
- **C.** universal life energy
- **D.** spirit

AP   **363.** Jin Shin Do is an oriental therapy that is
  A. preventative rather than symptomatic in nature
  B. to strengthen our absorption of life energy
  C. acupressure with breathing and meditation
  D. all of the above

P   **364.** A condition of the skin marked by elevations with clear fluid from contact with poison ivy is called a
  A. cyst
  B. vesicle
  C. macule
  D. laceration

AP   **365.** The Chinese consider the lung as the delicate organ because
  A. it is a delicate tissue
  B. it is the first organ to be injured by negative substances
  C. it cannot work without the heart
  D. all of the above

AP   **366.** Which type of muscle has striations, a single nucleus, intercalated discs, sarcomeres, transverse tubules, and gap junctions between fibers?
  A. Cardiac
  B. Multiunit smooth
  C. Skeletal
  D. Visceral smooth

AP   **367.** If a muscle is not used, the resulting condition is called
  A. atrophy
  B. rust
  C. hypertrophy
  D. myosin

AP   **368.** Which direction of muscle fiber is described as running parallel to the body's midline?
  A. Brevis
  B. Oblique
  C. Rectus abdominis
  D. Serratus

AP   **369.** Which facial muscle is the major cheek muscle?
- **A.** Buccinator
- **B.** Depressor labii inferioris
- **C.** Mentalis
- **D.** Platysma

AP   **370.** Describing how the organs or body parts function and relate to one another is the study of
- **A.** physiology
- **B.** histology
- **C.** anatomy
- **D.** pathology

AP   **371.** Which of the following abdominal muscles is **NOT** located in the anterior part of the abdomen?
- **A.** External oblique
- **B.** Internal oblique
- **C.** Quadratus lumborum
- **D.** Rectus abdominis

AP   **372.** At which vertebral level does the spinal cord end?
- **A.** First lumbar
- **B.** Between first and second lumbar
- **C.** Fifth lumbar
- **D.** Second sacral

AP   **373.** Which of the following is **NOT** a functional component of a reflex arc?
- **A.** Brain
- **B.** Effector
- **C.** Motor neuron
- **D.** Receptor

AP   **374.** Which reflex is essential to maintaining muscle tone and adjusts muscle performance during exercise?
- **A.** Crossed extensor
- **B.** Flexor
- **C.** Stretch
- **D.** Tendon

AP   **375.** Smooth muscles contract
- **A.** involuntarily
- **B.** forcefully
- **C.** voluntarily
- **D.** occasionally

AP   **376.** The deltoid muscle abducts the arm, and is often used as a site of injection. Which nerve stimulates it?
- **A.** Axillary
- **B.** Median
- **C.** Musculocutaneous
- **D.** Radial

P   **377.** Cancer is a disease that can be spread through the
- **A.** genes
- **B.** lymphatic and blood system
- **C.** endocrine system
- **D.** digestive system

P   **378.** Weak thumb movements, pain in the palm and fingers, and an inability to pronate the forearm are characteristics of an injury to which nerve?
- **A.** Median
- **B.** Medial pectoral
- **C.** Musculocutaneous
- **D.** Radial

AP   **379.** The sciatic nerve is actually two nerves. Which nerves compose the sciatic nerve?
- **A.** Common peroneal and pudendal
- **B.** Tibial and medial plantar
- **C.** Medial and lateral plantars
- **D.** Common peroneal and tibial

AP   **380.** Which of the following are involved in the abduction of the arm?
- **A.** Deltoid and subscapularis
- **B.** Supraspinatus and infraspinatus
- **C.** Teres major and teres minor
- **D.** Supraspinatus and deltoid

AP   **381.** Which of the following are involved in the adduction of the arm?
      A. Pectoralis major and latissimus dorsi
      B. Infraspinatus and teres major
      C. Teres minor and coracobrachialis
      D. Pectoralis major, teres major, teres minor, latissimus dorsi, carica brachialis

M   **382.** The Trager method uses movement exercises called
      A. gymnastics
      B. mentastics
      C. spirals
      D. athletics

P   **383.** Massage is **NOT** performed on an area that is
      A. bleeding
      B. swollen
      C. burned
      D. all of the above

AP   **384.** Which of the following is **NOT** part of the erector spinae muscles?
      A. Iliocostalis
      B. Longissimus
      C. Spinalis
      D. Platysma

AP   **385.** Which of the following muscles does **NOT** abduct the thigh?
      A. Gluteus maximus
      B. Gluteus medius
      C. Gluteus minimus
      D. Sartorius

AP   **386.** Which of the following laterally rotates the thigh?
      A. Obturator externus
      B. Obturator internus
      C. Piriformis
      D. All of the above

AP **387.** Blood is supplied to the forehead by the
- **A.** temporal artery
- **B.** facial artery
- **C.** frontal artery
- **D.** aorta

AP **388.** Which of the following is the major muscle involved in crossing one's leg?
- **A.** Gastrocnemius
- **B.** Rectus femoris
- **C.** Sartorius
- **D.** Semimembranosis

P **389.** Local anesthetics, such as Novocaine, block pain and other sensations by
- **A.** distracting the signal to the brain
- **B.** numbing the blood vessels next to the cut
- **C.** preventing the voltage leakage channels from leaking
- **D.** preventing the opening of voltage-gated sodium channels

AP **390.** The Amma therapy is a full-body manipulation of the Co-etaneous Regions, twelve organ channels, governing and conception vessels as well as
- **A.** Tendino-Muscle Channels
- **B.** TS points
- **C.** Yin-Yang
- **D.** Qi of the Heaven

P **391.** Epilepsy is characterized by
- **A.** short, recurrent periodic attacks of motor, sensory, or psychological malfunction
- **B.** epileptic seizures, which are initiated by abnormal, synchronous electrical discharges from the brain
- **C.** a person often contracting skeletal muscles involuntarily
- **D.** all of the above

AP 392. Which of the following statements about synaptic facts is **FALSE**?
   A. At a chemical synapse, only synaptic end bulbs of presynaptic neurons can release neurotransmitters
   B. Electrical synapses allow faster communication than do chemical synapses
   C. At a chemical synapse, ionic current spreads directly from one cell to another through gap junctions
   D. Presynaptic facilitation increases the amount of neurotransmitters released by a presynaptic neuron, whereas presynaptic inhibition decreases it

AP 393. Which cranial nerve is correctly paired with its number?
   A. Olfactory – I
   B. Trigeminal – V
   C. Facial – X
   D. Vestibulocochlear – VIII

AP 394. Which muscles help to stabilize the scapula for movement of the arms?
   A. Serratus anterior/rhomboids
   B. Rhomboids/gluteals
   C. Triceps/trapezius
   D. Pectoralis major/serratus anterior

P 395. Which of the following is **TRUE** about headaches?
   A. Analgesic and tranquilizing compounds are generally not effective for migraine headaches
   B. Migraines have been found to be helped by drugs that constrict the blood vessels
   C. Tension headaches classically occur in the occipital and temporal muscles
   D. All of the above

P 396. When massage is used to relieve muscle fatigue, it works mainly on the
   A. digestive system
   B. circulatory system
   C. endocrine system
   D. integumentary system

AP **397.** Which of the following brain areas are thought to be associated with memory?
  A. Frontal lobe and temporal lobe association cortex
  B. Occipital lobe and parietal lobe association cortex
  C. Parts of the limbic system and diencephalon
  D. All of the above

AP **398.** The major role for initiating and controlling precise, discrete muscular movements comes from the
  A. center of the thalamus
  B. bulk of the hypothalamus
  C. area lateral to the septum pellicidum
  D. motor portions of the cerebral cortex

P **399.** Loss of function of an entire arm is due to injury of the
  A. ulnar nerve
  B. median nerve
  C. radial nerve
  D. brachial plexus

P **400.** A ringing, roaring, or clicking in the ears is known as
  A. keratitis
  B. mydriasis
  C. scotoma
  D. tinnitus

P **401.** Conjunctivitis is
  A. a defect of vision
  B. an inflammation of the conjunctiva
  C. an inflammation of the auditory canal
  D. complete color blindness

AP **402.** An energy-balancing therapy that attempts to remove blockages and bring healing energy to the problem area is called
  A. reflexology
  B. therapeutic touch
  C. Amma therapy
  D. myofascial release

AP **403.** Which is an exocrine gland?
  - **A.** Pancreas
  - **B.** Thyroid
  - **C.** Salivary
  - **D.** Pituitary

AP **404.** Which of the following is characteristic of the sympathetic nervous system?
  - **A.** Heart rate decrease
  - **B.** Pupils constrict
  - **C.** Liver splits glycogen to glucose
  - **D.** Bronchioles constrict

AP **405.** What areas of the hypothalamus control the sympathetic division of the ANS?
  - **A.** Anterior and lateral
  - **B.** Anterior and medial
  - **C.** Posterior and medial
  - **D.** Posterior and lateral

AP **406.** Which part of the brain regulates the balance of sympathetic versus parasympathetic activity?
  - **A.** Hypothalamus
  - **B.** Medulla
  - **C.** Pineal gland
  - **D.** Pons

AP **407.** When the dorsum of the foot is massaged, which meridians are stimulated?
  - **A.** HT and KI
  - **B.** LIV and SP
  - **C.** LIV and ST
  - **D.** All Yang meridians

AP **408.** The cell body for the ANS's postganglionic neuron is in
  - **A.** the sensory root
  - **B.** an autonomic ganglion
  - **C.** the dorsal root ganglion
  - **D.** the brain or spinal cord

AP **409.** Glucagon
　　A. accelerates the formation of glycogen from glucose (glycogenesis)
　　B. promotes glucose formation from lactate and certain amino acids
　　C. lowers the blood glucose level
　　D. does all of the above functions

AP **410.** Which of the following is **NOT** produced by the ovary?
　　A. Androgen
　　B. Estrogen
　　C. Inhibin
　　D. Progesterone

AP **411.** The calcaneus is commonly known as the
　　A. ankle
　　B. knee
　　C. heel
　　D. elbow

AP **412.** Which of the following is **TRUE** about oxytocin (OT)?
　　A. It is secreted by the anterior pituitary gland
　　B. It is used as part of the birth control pill
　　C. It is inhibited by progesterone
　　D. Its synthetic form is known as prostaglandin

AP **413.** Which of the following is **TRUE** about antidiuretic hormone (ADH)?
　　A. During dehydration, ADH increases the rate of perspiration production
　　B. Alcohol stimulates ADH secretion
　　C. Pain, trauma, and anxiety suppress the secretion of ADH
　　D. It is also called vasopressin

AP **414.** The blood type that is termed the "universal donor" is
　　A. O
　　B. A
　　C. B
　　D. AB

B/E **415.** If you are not going to be a self-employed massage therapist, you might work for a
- **A.** cruise ship
- **B.** resort hotel
- **C.** chiropractor
- **D.** all of the above

AP **416.** The Jin Shin Do "middle way" of finger pressure is
- **A.** an application of pressure more than Ki
- **B.** feeling the hardness of the muscle
- **C.** below the epidermal touch
- **D.** all of the above

P **417.** A stationary clot in an unbroken vessel is called a (an)
- **A.** thrombus
- **B.** embolus
- **C.** fibulous
- **D.** prostaglandin

P **418.** An elevation of basophils in the body may be the result of
- **A.** burns
- **B.** parasitic infection
- **C.** leukemias and cancer
- **D.** high steroid levels

AP **419.** Blood pressure is lowest in
- **A.** veins
- **B.** capillaries
- **C.** arteries
- **D.** arterioles

AP **420.** The ability of a cell to engulf foreign matter is termed
- **A.** kinocytosis
- **B.** pinocytosis
- **C.** diapedesis
- **D.** phagocytosis

P **421.** An abnormally high percentage of red blood cells is termed
- **A.** erythrocythemia
- **B.** hypererythrocythemia
- **C.** polycythemia
- **D.** hypocythemia

AP   **422.** The process of erythrocyte formation is called
- **A.** hemopoiesis
- **B.** reticulopoiesis
- **C.** erythropoiesis
- **D.** chemopoiesis

P   **423.** A lower-than-normal number of RBCs is termed
- **A.** hypoxia
- **B.** erythropoietin
- **C.** normoblastin
- **D.** anemia

M   **424.** In oriental theory, Yin energy flows
- **A.** anterior to posterior
- **B.** dorsal to ventral
- **C.** inferior to superior
- **D.** superior to inferior

AP   **425.** A biconcave shaped cell that is 7 microns wide and that lacks a nucleus and cannot reproduce is a
- **A.** monocyte
- **B.** erythrocyte
- **C.** leukocyte
- **D.** thrombocyte

AP   **426.** Plasma constitutes what percentage of the blood?
- **A.** 20%
- **B.** 40%
- **C.** 55%
- **D.** 45%

AP   **427.** Which of the following is (are) **NOT** a formed element?
- **A.** Neutrophils
- **B.** T-cells
- **C.** Globulin
- **D.** Monocytes

AP   **428.** Blood carries
- **A.** carbon dioxide
- **B.** metabolic waste
- **C.** oxygen
- **D.** all of the above

AP   **429.** Which of the following is (are) functions of the blood?
- **A.** Transportation
- **B.** Regulation
- **C.** Protection
- **D.** All of the above

M   **430.** Practitioners use joint movements for a variety of reasons including
- **A.** to stretch surrounding tissue
- **B.** to increase range of motion
- **C.** to increase kinesthetic awareness
- **D.** all of the above

AP   **431.** In the middle of the thoracic cavity is a space assigned to the heart called the
- **A.** pleural space
- **B.** pericardial space
- **C.** mediastinum
- **D.** sternal notch

AP   **432.** A group of nerve cells that lie outside the CNS is called
- **A.** gray matter
- **B.** white matter
- **C.** ganglion
- **D.** nucleus

AP   **433.** Shortly after childbirth, the ductus arteriosus closes, leaving the remnant known as the
- **A.** ligamentum arteriosum
- **B.** ductus venosus
- **C.** coronary ligaments
- **D.** fossa ovalis

AP   **434.** The pulmonary circulation carries deoxygenated blood from the right ventricle to the air sacs of the lungs and returns oxygenated blood from the lungs to the
- **A.** right atrium
- **B.** left ventricle
- **C.** left atrium
- **D.** pulmonary valve

AP   **435.** The first and largest branch of the arch of the aorta is the
- **A.** subclavian
- **B.** coronary
- **C.** carotid
- **D.** brachiocephalic

M   **436.** Connective tissue massage (CTM) is a useful technique for
- **A.** preparing for surgery
- **B.** psychoemotional status
- **C.** loosening tissue following surgery or trauma
- **D.** controlling pain

AP   **437.** Within the brain, all veins drain into the
- **A.** external jugular veins
- **B.** internal jugular veins
- **C.** vertebral veins
- **D.** cardiac veins

P   **438.** A rapid resting heart or pulse rate over 100 beats per minute is termed
- **A.** bradycardia
- **B.** myocardia
- **C.** pericardia
- **D.** tachycardia

AP   **439.** Besides the heart, which of the following structures act as a pump to boost venous return?
- **A.** Smooth muscles and the diaphragm
- **B.** Skeletal muscles of the leg and diaphragm
- **C.** Skeletal muscles of the leg and smooth muscles
- **D.** Smooth muscles and changes in the thorax and abdomen

AP   **440.** Blood vessels that always carry blood away from the heart and usually carry oxygen are
- **A.** veins
- **B.** venules
- **C.** arteries
- **D.** capillaries

M 441. Skeletal muscle is affected by massage for which of the following symptoms?
    A. Increased muscle tension
    B. Muscle injury
    C. Spasm or cramp
    D. All of the above

AP 442. Lymph in the right leg would drain into the
    A. right lymphatic duct
    B. left thoracic duct
    C. cisterna chyli
    D. B and C are correct

AP 443. The spleen functions in all the following ways **EXCEPT**
    A. filtering of lymph
    B. site of B cell proliferation
    C. phagocytosis of bacteria and old RBCs
    D. stores and releases blood on demand

AP 444. Lymph is **MOST** similar to which of the following?
    A. Whole blood
    B. Blood plasma
    C. Interstitial fluid
    D. Intracellular fluid

AP 445. The pancreatic duct joins the common bile duct from the liver and gallbladder, and enters the duodenum at the
    A. ampulla of vater
    B. hepatopancreatic ampulla
    C. hepatic ampulla
    D. both A and B

B/E 446. SOAP charting is being widely adopted by massage professionals because
    A. use of a professional reporting system enhances the image of massage as a valuable therapy
    B. other health care professionals cannot understand the language
    C. it can be used in a court of law
    D. clients want a record of their health

AP **447.** The Yin and Yang comprise a spiral of change that represents
  A. seasons
  B. life in constant flux
  C. rhythms in animals and man
  D. all of the above

M **448.** The reflex effects of massage are the stimulation of
  A. motor neurons
  B. sensory receptors of skin and subcutaneous tissues
  C. synovial fluid at each joint
  D. chemotransmitter

AP **449.** Which of the following elements or nutrients is (are) the body's preferred source for synthesizing ATP?
  A. Glucose
  B. Fructose
  C. Amino acids
  D. Acetyl coenzyme A

AP **450.** The end product of glycolysis is pyruvic acid, and its fate depends on
  A. the body cellular need
  B. the availability of oxygen
  C. the transport in the bloodstream
  D. all of the above

Practice Test Questions 3

Answers and Discussion

301. (D) Massage therapy is used for whiplash, delivery, neuritis, and neuralgia. *(Ref. 9, p. 27)*

302. (A) Lymph fluid consists of water, cell debris, gases, metabolic waste, and bacteria. *(Ref. 2, p. 542)*

303. (D) The right thoracic duct is the correct place to start lymph massage. *(Ref. 2, pp. 544–547)*

304. (D) Business expenses include the costs of license, insurance, cards, linens and professional clothes, and memberships. *(Ref. 4, p. 84)*

305. (D) Client files document all the work you have done for your use and for the IRS. *(Ref. 4, p. 80)*

306. (D) Legitimate tax deductions are part of good records and bookkeeping. *(Ref. 4, p. 82)*

307. (D) If self-employed, you must file the 1040 IRS Form and Social Security Self-Employment Tax Form. *(Ref. 4, p. 88)*

308. (D) Marketing includes business cards and brochures, publications, and presentations. *(Ref. 4, pp. 114–117)*

309. (B) Good records should include intake and health information and session notes. *(Ref. 4, pp. 208–211)*

310. (B) All important information should be included on intake: name, address, phone, and physician. *(Ref. 4, p. 209)*

311. (B) Any psychological effects on a person cannot be inhibited by massage. *(Ref. 5, p. 4)*

312. (D) A lubricant avoids an uncomfortable friction on the skin of the patient. *(Ref. 5, p. 14)*

313. (D) Business deductions include something that helps to develop or maintain your trade including equipment, rent, phone, and any professional fees. *(Ref. 10, p. 125)*

314. (D) A systemic inflammation occurs when an irritant spreads through the body and becomes chronic, such as asthma, arthritis and bronchitis. *(Ref. 11, p. 92)*

315. (B) The removal of dead skin is a benefit of massage. *(Ref. 5, p. 33)*

316. (C) The brain releases endorphins, which act as pain relievers when stimulated by massage. *(Ref. 5, p. 45)*

317. (D) Mennell's stroke is unique since it goes only in one direction, with the hand returning in the air. *(Ref. 5, p. 74)*

318. (A) Relaxation results from the effleurage stroke. *(Ref. 5, p. 69)*

319. (C) When the muscle is "milked," the blood is returned to the heart via the venous return. *(Ref. 5, p. 77)*

320. (B) The history intake of an abused client sets up mental and physical limits and reassures the client that you will be understanding. *(Ref. 10, p. 81)*

321. (D) The urinary system regulates the chemical composition of the blood. *(Ref. 8, p. 18)*

322. **(A)** Contralateral is lateral on the opposite side of the body. *(Ref. 8, p. 15)*

323. **(D)** The movement of connective tissue is known as myofascial therapy designed by John Barnes and John Upledger. *(Ref. 11, p. 367)*

324. **(C)** The teres major is not part of the SITS muscles of the rotator cuff. It is located on the scapula and humerus for rotation and extension. *(Ref. 3, p. 47)*

325. **(C)** The nervous and endocrine systems respond to homeostatic responses. *(Ref. 8, p. 10)*

326. **(D)** Pain is difficult to explain or describe because it is a complex of symptoms that include psychological, social, and physiological aspects. *(Ref. 11, p. 2)*

327. **(D)** The office location requires that you meet the local governmental requirements including application for new business, zoning, and fire and health inspection. *(Ref. 10, p. 55)*

328. **(D)** Water is the most abundant inorganic molecule. *(Ref. 8, p. 37)*

329. **(D)** The pH of 6 is considered an acidic pH compared to water at 7. *(Ref. 8, p. 39)*

330. **(A)** The lymph capillaries form small valves allowing lymph to flow in one direction into larger lymph vessels. *(Ref. 2, p. 184)*

331. **(A)** Only the trapezium is stretched with a lateral flexation of the neck. *(Ref. 5, p. 111)*

332. **(D)** The Yin of the muscle channels passes through the muscles of the forearm, arm, shoulder, and chest. *(Ref. 12, p. 94)*

333. **(B)** A 10% bleach solution is the clean-up for HIV, hepatitis, and viral organisms. The solution is one cup bleach to one gallon of water. *(Ref. 11, p. 115)*

334. **(D)** Carbon dioxide and water are the end products of glucose. *(Ref. 8, p. 42)*

335. **(A)** Antibodies are proteins produced by the immune system that are stimulated through massage and act on specific antigens. *(Ref. 2, p. 187)*

336. **(A)** All the Yang channels meet with the deep and superficial pathways of the Governing Vessels at GV1 to GV28. *(Ref. 12, p. 93)*

337. **(B)** The massage therapist will move away from the client when the massage is complete so that it is understood that the session is over. *(Ref. 11, p. 35)*

338. **(D)** The mast cells comprise connective tissue that produces histamine. *(Ref. 8, p. 108)*

339. **(D)** The outermost layer of the skin is epidermis, composed of stratified squamous epithelium. *(Ref. 8, p. 138)*

340. **(C)** One of the aging factors is a decrease in fibroblasts. *(Ref. 8, p. 138)*

341. **(D)** Sunburn has been classified as a first-degree burn. *(Ref. 8, p. 139)*

342. **(A)** In second-degree burns, the epidermis and possibly the dermis are damaged. *(Ref. 8, p. 139)*

343. **(D)** Client assessment includes a history, observation, and an examination. *(Ref. 2, p. 295)*

344. **(A)** Ingham developed her method of *Zone Therapy* called reflexology and started to teach about healing the body by pressing the feet. *(Ref. 5, p. 234)*

345. **(D)** The bone matrix is hard due to the primary salt of calcium chloride. *(Ref. 8, p. 149)*

346. **(D)** When the radius is fractured on the distal end, it is classified as a Colle's fracture. *(Ref. 8, p. 156)*

347. **(A)** Erosion of the articular cartilage resulting in the bones touching is diagnosed as osteoarthritis. *(Ref. 2, p. 101; Ref. 8, p. 162)*

348. **(D)** Condyles are on the ends of long bones and form the joint of an articulation. *(Ref. 8, p. 167)*

349. (B) When assessing passive movement, the springy end feel is the most common. The end feel indicates the presence, type, and severity of lesions in the tissue associated with the joint. *(Ref. 2, p. 437)*

350. (B) The cranial bones in the skull contain two paired bones: the parietal and temporal. *(Ref. 8, p. 173)*

351. (D) The trochlea of the humerus articulates with the ulna. *(Ref. 8, p. 202)*

352. (C) The medial malleolus is the ankle bone projection on the medial side. *(Ref. 8, p. 211)*

353. (A) The tarsal bones include the calcaneus or heel for the Achille's tendon attachment. *(Ref. 8, p. 212)*

354. (C) The diarthrosis joints are classified as freely movable, including the ball and socket, hinges, and pivot. *(Ref. 8, p. 226)*

355. (D) The thumb is classified with a saddle joint for movement at the carpal and metacarpal articulation. *(Ref. 8, p. 226)*

356. (D) The single hinge of the knee and elbow and the double hinge of the wrist and ankle are types of diarthroses joints. *(Ref. 8, p. 226)*

357. (A) The knee contains many ligaments that are intraarticular and include the ACL (anterior cruciate ligament). *(Ref. 8, p. 232)*

358. (A) Damage to the anterior cruciate ligament of the knee is a very common injury in accidents involving the knee joint. *(Ref. 8, p. 230)*

359. (B) Neurons do not repair at all when the nervous system is injured or traumatized. *(Ref. 2, p. 40)*

360. (D) Skeletal muscles are the only type of muscle cells that are multinucleated. *(Ref. 8, p. 238)*

361. (C) With every physiological problem there is always a psychological ramification; there is a never-ending interaction between the mind and the body. *(Ref. 12, p. 12)*

362. (C) Ki within the universe is used within our bodies as a purification or toxification unit for this energy. *(Ref. 13, p. 30)*

363. (D) Jin Shin Do developed as a preventative health art to strengthen the absorption of Ki through acupressure, meditation, and breathing. *(Ref. 13, p. 14, 30)*

364. (B) Vesicles are blisters with clear fluid that lie just beneath the epidermis. *(Ref. 2, p. 79; Ref. 8, p. 5)*

365. (B) The lung generally is the first line of exposure and defense by a negative substance or energy and has been identified as the delicate organ. *(Ref. 12, pp. 110–111)*

366. (A) The characteristics of the cardiac muscle tissue include intercalated discs, striations, single nucleus, gap junction, and transverse tubules. *(Ref. 8, p. 263)*

367. (A) Atrophy is a condition in which the muscle cannot be contracted or is very weakened and begins to waste away. *(Ref. 2, p. 123)*

368. (C) Abdominis muscle runs adjacent to the midline in a parallel direction. *(Ref. 8, p. 272)*

369. (A) The major cheek muscle is the buccinator, which is able to compress and blow out in the sucking motion. *(Ref. 8, p. 279)*

370. (A) Physiology is the study of vital processes and functions of body parts. *(Ref. 2, p. 35)*

371. (C) The quadratus lumborum is a small muscle in the posterior part of the abdomen located on the lumbar vertebrae and T12. *(Ref. 8, p. 294)*

372. (B) The spinal cord in the adult ends between the first and second lumbar vertebrae, which is called *conus medullaris*. *(Ref. 8, p. 376)*

373. (A) The reflex arc does not include the brain in the rapid adjustments to homeostatic balancing. Only the spinal cord integrates the reflex action. *(Ref. 8, p. 384)*

374. (C) The stretch reflex is important to maintaining and adjusting muscle tone through a monosynaptic reflex arc, one motor and one sensory. *(Ref. 8, p. 384)*

375. (A) The involuntary action of the smooth muscle is controlled by the autonomic nervous system maintaining long slow contractions. *(Ref. 2, p. 105)*

376. (A) The axillary nerve of the brachial plexus stimulates the deltoid muscle, which is used as an injection site. *(Ref. 8, p. 395)*

377. (B) The spreading of cancer or metastasis occurs through the blood or lymphatic system. *(Ref. 2, p. 258)*

378. (A) Median nerve damage affects thumb movement and the inability to flex the wrist and pronate the arm. *(Ref. 8, p. 394)*

379. (D) The sciatic nerve of the sacral plexus is composed of the common peroneal and tibial nerves arising from L4–S4. *(Ref. 8, p. 399)*

380. (D) The abduction of the humerus is accomplished by the deltoid muscle of the shoulder and the supraspinatus. *(Ref. 8, p. 305)*

381. (D) The adduction of the arm is accomplished by the pectoralis major of the chest, teres major, latissimus dorsi, and the brachialis. *(Ref. 8, p. 305)*

382. (B) Mentastics is the gentle rocking or shaking of body parts, called the Trager method. *(Ref. 2, p. 16; Ref. 5, p. 299)*

383. (D) There are many contraindications to massage including bleeding, swelling, burns, skin infections, tumors, and bruises. *(Ref. 2, p. 259)*

384. (D) The erector spinae muscles are composed of three separate muscles: iliocostalis, longissimus, and spinalis. The platysma is found in the face. *(Ref. 8, pp. 318–321)*

385. (A) The gluteus maximus extends and rotates the thigh laterally. It does not abduct the thigh. *(Ref. 8, p. 323)*

386. (D) Lateral rotation of the thigh is accomplished by the deep muscles, including the obturator externus and internus, and piriformis. *(Ref. 8, p. 323)*

387. (C) A branch of the external carotid artery is the frontal artery that supplies the forehead. *(Ref. 2, p. 178)*

388. (C) The sartorius muscle is the longest muscle found in the leg and laterally rotates when crossing over the knee. *(Ref. 8, p. 330)*

389. (D) Anesthetics block pain so that nerve impulses cannot pass the obstructed region by preventing the opening of the sodium channels. *(Ref. 8, p. 361)*

390. (A) The Trendino-Muscle Channels are part of the full-body manipulation technique used by the Amma therapist to promote the flow of Qi, blood, and fluids. *(Ref. 12, p. 73)*

391. (D) The symptoms of epilepsy include seizures, involuntary muscle contraction, and short attacks of motor sensory or psychological malfunction. *(Ref. 8, p. 372)*

392. (C) The false statement is that at the chemical synapse ions do not travel through gap junctions. *(Ref. 8, p. 364)*

393. (D) The sense of hearing is the vestibulocochlear cranial nerve—VIII. *(Ref. 8, p. 412)*

394. (A) The rhomboids are attached from the scapula to the vertebrae, and they stabilize the arm movement along with the anterior serratus. *(Ref. 2, p. 122)*

395. (D) Headaches generally occur in the occipital and temporal muscle area. Migraines cannot be helped by analgesics but by drugs that can constrict the blood vessels. *(Ref. 8, p. 440)*

396. (B) Muscle fatigue is relieved by mechanical action on the blood vessels and massaging toward the heart. *(Ref. 2, pp. 250, 486)*

397. (D) The memory is associated with frontal temporal, occipital, and parietal lobe association cortex and parts of the limbic system and diencephalon. *(Ref. 8, p. 423)*

398. (D) The cerebral cortex has areas for muscle movement that are action-specific for motor movements. *(Ref. 8, p. 424)*

399. (D) The nerves of the brachial plexus control movement of the arm. *(Ref. 2, p. 199)*

400. (D) Tinnitus is described as the ringing or sounds in the ear as a result of high blood pressure or nerve degeneration. *(Ref. 8, p. 499)*

401. (B) An inflammation of the conjunctiva is pink eye, caused by bacteria, and is very contagious. *(Ref. 8, p. 499)*

402. (C) Amma therapy treats the body by assessing energy imbalances and dysfunctional organs and then brings healing energy to those areas. *(Ref. 12, p. 6)*

403. (C) The salivary gland is an exocrine gland because it is ducted. *(Ref. 2, p. 77)*

404. (C) The sympathetic nervous system is in control of promoting glycogen synthesis and increasing bile secretion. *(Ref. 8, p. 512)*

405. (D) The hypothalamus control of the sympathetic division of the ANS is posterior and lateral. *(Ref. 8, p. 505)*

406. (A) The hypothalamus part of the brain regulates the balance of sympathetic and parasympathetic activity. *(Ref. 8, p. 513)*

407. (B) The liver and spleen meridians are stimulated when the dorsum of the foot is massaged. *(Ref. 2, p. 566)*

408. (B) The cell body for the autonomic nervous system is the postganglionic neuron. *(Ref. 8, p. 507)*

409. (B) The hormone glucagon stimulates formation of glucose from lactate and amino acids. *(Ref. 8, p. 549)*

410. (A) The ovary produces and secretes the hormones estrogen and progesterone. Androgen is a male hormone. *(Ref. 8, p. 553)*

411. (C) The heel is the calcaneus bone. *(Ref. 3, p. 31)*

412. **(C)** In the female, the hormone progesterone inhibits the action of oxytocin. *(Ref. 8, p. 535)*

413. **(D)** Some hormones are known by alternate names, including vasopressin for ADH. *(Ref. 8, p. 534)*

414. **(A)** A person who is able to give blood to all other blood types has type O and is the universal donor. *(Ref. 8, p. 585)*

415. **(C)** Microscopic air sacs found in the lungs are called alveoli. *(Ref. 3, p. 96)*

416. **(D)** The erythrocyte contains blood type antigens and the Rh or D antigen. *(Ref. 8, p. 585)*

417. **(A)** When a blood clot remains stationary, it is called a thrombus. *(Ref. 8, p. 583)*

418. **(C)** In leukemia and cancer, the WBC increases. *(Ref. 8, p. 574)*

419. **(A)** There is no blood pressure in the veins as compared to the arteries. *(Ref. 2, p. 168)*

420. **(D)** When the cell attacks foreign material, the engulfing process is phagocytosis. *(Ref. 8, p. 576)*

421. **(C)** When the RBCs are higher than normal, the condition is called polycythemia, i.e., "too many." *(Ref. 8, p. 524)*

422. **(C)** The bone marrow functions as the site of blood cell production. Red blood cell development is called erythropoiesis. *(Ref. 8, p. 569)*

423. **(D)** When the RBCs drop below the normal number, the condition is known as anemia. *(Ref. 8, p. 568)*

424. **(C)** The flow of energy of Yin is from the inferior part of the body to the superior. *(Ref. 2, p. 564)*

425. **(B)** All blood cell types have a nucleus except the erythrocyte. The thrombocyte is only a cell fragment. *(Ref. 8, p. 570)*

426. (C) The liquid portion of the blood is plasma, which is 55% of the total volume. *(Ref. 8, p. 568)*

427. (C) The neutrophils, T-cells, and monocytes are formed elements. The globulins are proteins found in the blood. *(Ref. 8, p. 569)*

428. (D) The blood is the transport system for metabolic wastes, gases, nutrients, hormones, and salts. *(Ref. 8, p. 567)*

429. (D) The blood provides many functions to the body, including regulation of temperature, transport, and protection. *(Ref. 8, p. 567)*

430. (D) Movement of the joints stimulate muscle relaxation, increases ROM and kinesthetic awareness, as well as stretching surrounding tissue and stimulating production of synovial fluid. *(Ref. 5, p. 111)*

431. (C) The mediastinum is the medial part of the thoracic cavity containing the heart. *(Ref. 8, p. 592)*

432. (C) Ganglia are masses of neurons that extend along the outside of the spine and synapse with other neurons. *(Ref. 2, p. 196)*

433. (A) The mature heart contains the ligamentum arteriosum, which closes after birth. *(Ref. 8, p. 615)*

434. (C) In blood flow, the lungs return oxygenated blood to the left side of the heart at the atrium. *(Ref. 8, p. 673)*

435. (D) The aorta artery branches after it leaves the heart with the major brachiocephalic. *(Ref. 8, p. 648)*

436. (C) CTM improves circulation and postoperative ANS reflexes that increase sympathetic nerve activity. *(Ref. 9, p. 6)*

437. (B) The vena cava branches into the jugular vein, which drains the blood from the brain. *(Ref. 8, p. 663)*

438. (D) When there is a heartbeat more than 100 beats per minute, the result is tachycardia. *(Ref. 8, p. 630)*

439. (B) The skeletal muscles of the legs move the blood back to the heart. *(Ref. 8, p. 634)*

440. **(C)**   Arteries are the oxygen-rich vessels that carry blood away from the heart. *(Ref. 8, p. 624)*

441. **(D)**   The muscle responds to massage after an injury, spasm, or tension. *(Ref. 9, p. 10)*

442. **(D)**   Drainage of lymph from the right leg enters the cisterna chyli and then the left thoracic duct. *(Ref. 8, p. 686)*

443. **(A)**   The spleen destroys old RBCs, produces some lymphocytes, and can store and release blood. *(Ref. 8, p. 689)*

444. **(C)**   The interstitial fluid of the body drains into the lymphatic system. *(Ref. 8, p. 683)*

445. **(D)**   The ampulla of vater and hepatopancreatic ampulla enter the duodenum. *(Ref. 8, p. 788)*

446. **(A)**   SOAP charting is an efficient and effective way to document all types of health care treatment. *(Ref. 14, p. 8)*

447. **(D)**   To follow the Yin-Yang principle is to change from season to season, light to dark, warm to cold, and follow the continual rhythm of all life. *(Ref. 13, p. 23)*

448. **(B)**   Stimulation of the sensory receptors of the skin is the reflex effect of massage. *(Ref. 5, p. 33)*

449. **(A)**   Glucose enters the cell respiration to form molecules of ATP. *(Ref. 8, p. 825)*

450. **(D)**   An aerobic process converts glucose into pyruvic acid, provided a blood supply and oxygen are available. *(Ref. 8, p. 826)*

Practice Test Questions 4

CONTENT CODES

M = Massage and Bodywork   AP = Anatomy and Physiology
P = Pathology   B/E = Business/Ethics

DIRECTIONS: Each of the numbered items or incomplete statements in this chapter is followed by answers or completions of the statement. Select the **ONE** lettered answer or completion that is **BEST** in each case.

AP   **451.** The mineral that is found in the hemoglobin of blood and that carries oxygen to body cells is
   A. phosphorous
   B. calcium
   C. magnesium
   D. iron

P   **452.** A sore that has not healed properly is a warning sign for
   A. colds
   B. cancer
   C. flu
   D. mumps

P 453. The artificial cleansing and excretion of waste products from the blood is properly termed
A. hemodialysis
B. blood clearance
C. kidney evacuation
D. membrane indwelling

AP 454. The Qi pathways or channels constitute the
A. Shiatsu vessels
B. Amma bioenergy system
C. blood vessels
D. Chinese meridians

AP 455. Urine passes, in the order given, through which of the following structures?
A. Glomerulus, urethra, bladder, ureter
B. Hilum, bladder, ureter
C. Pelvis, ureter, bladder, urethra
D. Hilum, urethra, bladder, ureter

AP 456. The nephron is considered to be the
A. largest component of the kidney
B. vascular component of the urinary system
C. least necessary component of the kidney
D. functional unit of the kidney

P 457. Cardiac conditions, diabetes, lung disease, and high or low blood pressure are examples of contraindicators for
A. hydrotherapy
B. complications
C. side effects
D. benefits

AP 458. The five elements of fire, earth, metal, water, and wood are associated with
A. a five-pointed star
B. organs of the body
C. emotions, seasons, and climates
D. all of the above

AP **459.** The primary method of water movement into and out of body compartments is
- **A.** diffusion
- **B.** osmosis
- **C.** filtration
- **D.** hydrosis

M **460.** Ice massage is effective for local pain and
- **A.** swelling
- **B.** relaxed muscles
- **C.** fever
- **D.** systemic pain

AP **461.** The nucleus of a somatic cell contains the diploid chromosome number, symbolized 2n. In humans, this number is
- **A.** 23
- **B.** 12
- **C.** 46
- **D.** 30

M **462.** Nutrition is an important component to the therapist's wellness training because
- **A.** food dictates a work schedule
- **B.** without sugar, therapy is not possible
- **C.** diet affects the behavior and mood changes
- **D.** without fat in a diet the therapist can't stay warm

M **463.** Planning single and multiple client sessions
- **A.** is not easy to accomplish initially
- **B.** depends on the client history and interview
- **C.** depends on the emotional status of the client
- **D.** can only be effective after six visits

P **464.** Dysfunction caused by physical trauma or strain is associated with the
- **A.** autonomic nervous system
- **B.** sympathetic nervous system
- **C.** pain-spasm-pain cycle
- **D.** parasympathetic nervous system

M   **465.** The adhesions of a well-healed scar can be broken down between skin tissue by applying
    A. vibration
    B. petrissage
    C. friction
    D. effleurage

AP   **466.** A deficiency of this vitamin results in defective utilization of calcium by bones, which leads to rickets in children and osteomalacia in adults. This vitamin is
    A. vitamin E
    B. biotin
    C. vitamin K
    D. vitamin D

M   **467.** Massage of the lower extremity includes all but
    A. lying down with the leg in neutral position
    B. foot in 90° of dorsiflexion
    C. avoiding any massage around the knee
    D. not stroking too high on medial thigh

AP   **468.** The hormone that aids in determining the basal metabolic rate (BMR) is
    A. estrogen
    B. thyroid hormone
    C. insulin
    D. epinephrine

AP   **469.** According to the 12 meridians, vital energy, circulation, and nutrients flow start in the
    A. gall bladder (GB)
    B. liver (LIV)
    C. lung (L)
    D. pericardium (P)

P   **470.** Which of the following causes an increase in body temperature?
    A. Thyroid hormones
    B. Increased body production of epinephrine and norepinephrine into the blood
    C. Skeletal muscles contraction
    D. All of the above

P   **471.** Acquired immune deficiency syndrome (AIDS) is caused by HIV, which is an acronym for
      A. having the immune virus
      B. hapten immune virus
      C. human immune virus
      D. human immunodeficiency virus

AP   **472.** The average normal volume of blood in an adult is about
      A. 10 liters
      B. 5 liters
      C. 3 liters
      D. 2 liters

M   **473.** Reflexology of the hands and feet is based on
      A. polarity
      B. Traeger
      C. zone therapy
      D. hydrotherapy

AP   **474.** Which of the following is classified as a dense connective tissue?
      A. Adipose connective tissue
      B. Areolar connective tissue
      C. Elastic connective tissue
      D. Hyaline cartilage

AP   **475.** Which of the following is **TRUE** concerning cartilage?
      A. Except for that in the perichondrium, cartilage has no blood vessels or nerves
      B. The cells of mature cartilage are known as lacunae
      C. The resilience of cartilage is due to its collagen fiber
      D. There are three kinds of cartilage: hyaline, mosaic, and elastic

AP   **476.** You have a headache and rub your temple area immediately posterior to the zygomatic part of the orbit. You are rubbing the skin, connective tissue, and muscle over which bone?
      A. Frontal
      B. Parietal
      C. Sphenoid
      D. Temporal

P   **477.** Which term means an exaggeration of the lumbar curve of the vertebral column?
- **A.** Lordosis
- **B.** Kyphosis
- **C.** Scoliosis
- **D.** Spina bifida

AP   **478.** The axis is a special
- **A.** lumbar vertebra
- **B.** thoracic vertebra
- **C.** cervical vertebra
- **D.** sacral bone

AP   **479.** Which of the following is **TRUE** concerning the scapula?
- **A.** The end of the spine projects as the expanded process called the coracoid
- **B.** The coracoid articulates with the clavicle
- **C.** The glenoid cavity is where the scapula and humerus articulate
- **D.** The lateral border of the scapula is near the vertebral column

AP   **480.** What percentage of your body weight is due to your muscles?
- **A.** 10–20
- **B.** 20–30
- **C.** 30–40
- **D.** 40–50

P   **481.** The symptoms of an upper respiratory infection including bronchitis, cold, and sinusitis can benefit from
- **A.** light massage to area
- **B.** tapotement on the chest
- **C.** friction to the pectoral muscles
- **D.** slapping on the back

AP   **482.** Which of the following receptors help to monitor and control heart rate?
- **A.** Proprioceptors
- **B.** Chemoreceptors
- **C.** Baroreceptors
- **D.** All of the above

AP **483.** The exchange of oxygen and carbon dioxide between tissue blood capillaries and tissue cells is called
A. external respiration
B. pulmonary respiration
C. internal respiration
D. postpleural respiration

M **484.** A first-aid procedure designed to clear the air passageways of obstructing objects is known as the
A. pneumonectomy
B. Cheyne-Stokes
C. cardiopulmonary resuscitation
D. Heimlich maneuver

P **485.** A chronic, inflammatory disorder that produces sporadic narrowing of airways with periods of coughing, difficult breathing, and wheezing is called
A. asthma
B. bronchitis
C. emphysema
D. tuberculosis

B/E **486.** A ledger that separates and classifies every business expenditure is called a (an)
A. inventory
B. disbursement record
C. voucher
D. tax ID

B/E **487.** A record of monies owed to you by others is called
A. charges
B. accounts receivable
C. statements
D. liabilities

B/E **488.** Money that you owe to others is called
A. accounts payable
B. accounts receivable
C. assets
D. liabilities

B/E   **489.** Business activities directed toward promoting and increasing business are called
   A. assets
   B. reputation
   C. marketing
   D. goals

B/E   **490.** Developing personal and professional contacts for the purpose of giving and receiving support and sharing information is called
   A. hotline
   B. networking
   C. advertising
   D. promotions

B/E   **491.** A short, general statement of the business' main focus is called a (an)
   A. goal
   B. plan
   C. advertisement
   D. mission statement

B/E   **492.** A business that has stockholders is called a
   A. sole proprietorship
   B. partnership
   C. corporation
   D. subsidiary

B/E   **493.** The insurance that covers costs of injuries occurring on your property and any resulting litigation is called
   A. disability
   B. liability
   C. homeowner's
   D. theft

B/E   **494.** Standards for acceptable and professional behavior are called
   A. rules
   B. ethics
   C. malpractice
   D. codes

M   **495.** Massage benefits the nervous system by
       A. improving skin tone
       B. eliminating waste material
       C. relieving pain
       D. stimulating muscles

M   **496.** Massage benefits the skin by
       A. relieving stiffness
       B. improving tone
       C. opening pores
       D. removing pimples

P   **497.** All of the following are local (regional) contraindications for massage **EXCEPT**
       A. recent burn
       B. undiagnosed lump
       C. open sore
       D. shock

AP   **498.** For complete absorption, the average meal requires about
       A. 4 hours
       B. 10 hours
       C. 12 hours
       D. none of the above statements is accurate

M   **499.** Moving a joint without assistance or resistance is called
       A. flexion
       B. range of motion
       C. extension
       D. free movement

M   **500.** The application of water (in any form) to the body for therapeutic purposes is called
       A. floating
       B. hydrotherapy
       C. therapy
       D. washing

M   **501.** A mildly stimulating effect is produced by
       A. body oils
       B. effervescent tablets
       C. salt rub
       D. bath salts

M   **502.** Application of liquid to the body by means of a sponge, cloth, or hand is called
   A. sponging
   B. shampoo
   C. bath
   D. spray

P   **503.** Somatic pain arises from stimulation of receptors in the skin or from stimulation of receptors in the
   A. viscera
   B. peritoneum
   C. brain
   D. muscle, joints, tendons, and fascia

M   **504.** Prolonged use of cold applications has which effect?
   A. Stimulating
   B. Energizing
   C. Depressing
   D. Heating

M   **505.** Expansion of blood vessels following cold application is called a (an)
   A. primary effect
   B. secondary effect
   C. afterthought
   D. energizer

M   **506.** Hot water temperature in hydrotherapy should not exceed
   A. 100°F
   B. 110°F
   C. 115°F
   D. 120°F

M   **507.** A salt bath is similar to bathing in
   A. a lake
   B. a whirlpool
   C. a sauna
   D. sea water

M **508.** Hot baths or showers may overwork the
- **A.** water heater
- **B.** sweat glands
- **C.** brain
- **D.** heart

M **509.** A full-body steam bath for the purpose of causing perspiration is called a
- **A.** Swedish bath
- **B.** Japanese spa
- **C.** Greek soak
- **D.** Russian bath

M **510.** Prolonged application of cold leads to a physical condition called
- **A.** iglooism
- **B.** hyperthermia
- **C.** hypothermia
- **D.** freezer burn

M **511.** A type of dry heat is a (an)
- **A.** ice cube
- **B.** microwave
- **C.** sauna
- **D.** fog

M **512.** Hydrotherapy is the therapeutic use of
- **A.** generators
- **B.** water
- **C.** lotion
- **D.** massage

AP **513.** Which, of the following would lead to water retention?
- **A.** Hypertension
- **B.** Hypoventilation
- **C.** Vomiting
- **D.** Diarrhea

M   **514.** Spray showers are effective means of
   A. calming nerves
   B. hydrotherapy
   C. moist heat and mild compression
   D. all of the above

M   **515.** Application of cold should be of short duration to prevent tissue injury from
   A. pain
   B. thawing
   C. freezing
   D. heat

M   **516.** To increase circulation to an injured area and promote healing, a therapist can alternate applications of
   A. vibration and friction
   B. feathering and kneading
   C. heat and cold
   D. percussion and feathering

M   **517.** Instead of using a commercial ice pack, put ice cubes into a
   A. wash cloth
   B. dish towel
   C. plastic bag
   D. bath tub

M   **518.** Itching, inflammation, sensitivity, or a stinging sensation are considered
   A. normal
   B. reasonable
   C. allergic reactions
   D. safe

M   **519.** A massage table should be stable, firm, and
   A. tall
   B. short
   C. wide
   D. comfortable

B/E   **520.** Before setting up a massage practice, an important goal is
        A. owning your own place
        B. setting target deadlines for yourself
        C. to working for free initially
        D. to taking a bank loan

M   **521.** The height of a massage table is determined by the
        A. height of the client
        B. weight of the client
        C. practitioner's height
        D. size of the room

B/E   **522.** It is best to market your business by advertising in the
        A. newspaper
        B. Yellow Pages
        C. direct mail
        D. all of the above

M   **523.** A general massage practitioner often finds a multiple-position table to be
        A. of no use
        B. a good investment
        C. poorly constructed
        D. extra durable

M   **524.** Avoid using which type of oil in massage?
        A. Sunflower
        B. Mineral
        C. Olive
        D. Apricot

M   **525.** An appropriate oil combination is
        A. sesame and almond
        B. sunflower and canola
        C. apricot and olive
        D. peanut and walnut

M   **526.** Body areas where caution should be used to avoid damaging underlying anatomical structures are called
        A. contraindications
        B. endangerment sites

     C. off limits

     D. inferior

B/E   **527.** When a practitioner performs a massage in the client's home, it is called

     A. outcall

     B. extra service

     C. in-service

     D. intrusion

M   **528.** The ideal Fahrenheit temperature for a massage room is

     A. 75°

     B. 60°

     C. 90°

     D. 85°

M   **529.** Avoid lighting that shines

     A. on the client's legs

     B. on the client's back

     C. on the client's hands

     D. into the client's eyes

P   **530.** Acute inflammation is a massage

     A. side-effect

     B. contraindication

     C. indication

     D. benefit

M   **531.** Working on an area close to an affected area often stimulates circulation and promotes

     A. healing

     B. blood pressure

     C. blood sugar

     D. respiration

M   **532.** Direct physical effects of massage techniques on the tissues they contact are called

     A. reflex effects

     B. pressure points

     C. physiological effects

     D. mechanical effects

M   **533.** Gentle stroking, light friction, and petrissage are techniques called
       A. stimulatory
       B. muscular
       C. psychological
       D. sedative

B/E   **534.** In a personal service business, hygiene and safety are especially important to
       A. the client
       B. the facility
       C. the practitioner
       D. everyone concerned

B/E   **535.** It is important for the massage practitioner to know the difference between sensuality and
       A. sensitivity
       B. sexuality
       C. common sense
       D. sympathy

B/E   **536.** Inappropriate sexual interactions can lead to
       A. consequences
       B. increased business
       C. unethical conduct
       D. a reliable reputation

P   **537.** Acupressure helps to assess location of pain through palpation of
       A. bony landmarks
       B. energy blockages
       C. craniosacral pulses
       D. all of the above

B/E   **538.** Answering a client in a factual but tactful manner is called
       A. honesty
       B. camouflage
       C. tact
       D. manners

B/E   **539.** The ability to set positive goals and put forth the energy
and effort required to achieve them is
   A. self-motivation
   B. self-preservation
   C. self-indulgence
   D. selfishness

B/E   **540.** Business success is the result of
   A. luck
   B. proper degrees
   C. preparation
   D. family support

B/E   **541.** Keep your knowledge current by
   A. attending seminars
   B. reading trade journals
   C. joining professional associations
   D. all of the above

B/E   **542.** An important aspect of business is a (an)
   A. reliable reputation
   B. quick deal
   C. impressive decor
   D. gossipy employee

B/E   **543.** Reputation is also established by working
   A. late night hours
   B. regular business hours
   C. briskly
   D. weekly

B/E   **544.** To practice good ethics is to be concerned about the wel-
fare of the public and individual clients, as well as your
personal and professional
   A. health
   B. reputation
   C. clothing
   D. diet

B/E **545.** An important part of ethics is to keep client communications
  A. repeated
  B. confidential
  C. written down
  D. recorded

B/E **546.** A professional will, when necessary, refer clients to
  A. medical professionals
  B. hairstylists
  C. restaurants
  D. trainers

B/E **547.** A professional business is kept
  A. clean
  B. cluttered
  C. unsanitary
  D. dirty

B/E **548.** Universal precautions are used when administering first aid because
  A. you have to assume that anyone receiving first aid potentially has infectious diseases
  B. HIV is transmitted by exposure to blood and other body fluids
  C. hepatitis and other pathogens are transmitted by exposure to blood and other body fluids
  D. all of the above

B/E **549.** Confidentiality of your client's records is required for many reasons. The primary reason is
  A. to protect yourself if sued by the client
  B. to ensure adequate information for insurance billing purposes
  C. professional ethics
  D. you were told to do so by your Swedish instructor

B/E **550.** The immediate first-aid actions required in treating an injured person are
  A. talk to the individual, determine if he or she is responsive
  B. if possible, position the individual on the back (unless vomiting)

C. call 911 or other EMS, giving the exact location with identifying landmarks, your phone number, nature of the injury, the condition of victim, what is being done, and any other circumstances

D. all of the above

B/E **551.** You are self-employed. How often do you have to make estimated tax payments?

A. Once a month

B. Annually, before December 31 of the tax year

C. You do not; just pay your taxes before April 15 when the return is due

D. Quarterly

B/E **552.** When administering first aid, your goal is to obtain all the necessary information related to the injury. You should conduct a primary survey of the situation, which includes

A. checking the ABCs: airway, breathing, circulation, and hemorrhaging

B. using universal precautions when administering any first aid

C. assessing the victim's immediate condition and any unforeseen problems

D. all of the above

M **553.** The application of moist heat is superior to that of dry heat because of

A. convection

B. conduction

C. conversion

D. the greenhouse effect

M **554.** Which of the following is a local effect of cold therapy?

A. Vasodilation

B. Increased circulation

C. Vasoconstriction

D. Increased local metabolism

M   **555.** The most beneficial use of alternate hot/cold (contrast) treatments is with
        A. acute muscle spasm
        B. chronic muscle spasm
        C. insulin-dependent diabetes
        D. acute fibromyalgia

M   **556.** Alternative methods of stress reduction and relaxation techniques include
        A. breathing techniques
        B. visualization
        C. biofeedback
        D. all of the above

B/E   **557.** In rescue breathing, which of the following is done?
        A. Tilt the head back and lift chin
        B. Pinch nose shut
        C. Seal lips around mouth with two full breaths
        D. All of the above

B/E   **558.** In adult CPR, the pulse is
        A. not checked
        B. checked at the wrist
        C. checked at side of neck
        D. checked behind knee

B/E   **559.** If a person is suffering from heat cramps,
        A. do not give liquid with caffeine or alcohol
        B. do not give any medication
        C. cool with compresses at neck, groin, and armpits
        D. all of the above

B/E   **560.** In general heat exhaustion, heat stroke, and heat cramps require
        A. sleep
        B. liquids and shower
        C. cooling the victim and rest
        D. walking around to limber up

B/E **561.** The first-aid treatment for a seizure is aimed at
A. actively restoring consciousness
B. protecting victim from injury as it occurs
C. calming through massage
D. calling for help

B/E **562.** The first sign of a person choking is
A. pupils dilated
B. shallow breathing
C. victim cannot answer
D. coughing

B/E **563.** In CPR, the hands are placed on the
A. clavicle
B. posterior end of sternum
C. abdomen
D. pelvis

B/E **564.** To administer CPR, the victim must
A. not be breathing or have a pulse
B. be awake
C. be able to talk
D. be standing

B/E **565.** The universal distress signal of choking is
A. pointing to neck
B. rotating neck
C. clutching the neck between thumb and index finger
D. nodding the head

B/E **566.** The Heimlich maneuver is performed by
A. pressing the fist into the abdomen with inward thrust
B. subdiaphragmatic thrusts
C. standing behind victim with arms around waist
D. all of the above

B/E **567.** Signs of a stroke are
A. inability to eat or drink
B. old age
C. dizziness, numbness of the arm or leg on one side
D. thirst

M   **568.** In CPR performance, always
- **A.** pinch off the nostrils
- **B.** keep the head tilted
- **C.** watch for the victim's chest to rise
- **D.** all of the above

M   **569.** With an unconscious victim, always
- **A.** get a chair
- **B.** leave in any position
- **C.** turn victim on back if lying on a hard surface
- **D.** put pillow under head

M   **570.** A method to aid stress-related activities is
- **A.** wet compresses
- **B.** aerobics
- **C.** sleep
- **D.** deep breathing exercises

M   **571.** In massage, yoga enhances
- **A.** muscular control
- **B.** breathing
- **C.** relaxation
- **D.** all of the above

M   **572.** Meditation is a useful treatment for
- **A.** stimulating the flow of natural healing forces
- **B.** preventative treatment
- **C.** subliminal messages
- **D.** all of the above

P   **573.** Dr. Travell and Dr. Chaiton agree that gentle lengthening to reset the normal resting length of the muscle must follow therapy using
- **A.** polarity
- **B.** kinesiology
- **C.** trigger points
- **D.** meridians

M   **574.** The points to check while practicing massage are
- **A.** good body positioning and height
- **B.** comfort and relaxation of the patient
- **C.** even pressure throughout each stroke
- **D.** all of the above

M 575. Variations of effleurage include
    A. knuckling and stroking
    B. backstroke and friction
    C. pressure and brushing
    D. wide angling and stroking

M 576. Variations of petrissage include
    A. one-handed petrissage
    B. open and closed C position
    C. V hand position
    D. all of the above

M 577. In the application of the universal precautions issued by the CDC in 1987, massage therapists should avoid contact with
    A. blood
    B. vomit
    C. urine and feces
    D. all of the above

M 578. Variations of friction to mobilize the tissue under the skin is (are)
    A. wringing and squeezing
    B. knuckling and backstroke
    C. "hook on" stroke
    D. cross-fiber manipulation

M 579. The muscle or group that is not included in a massage of the back is
    A. trapezius
    B. rhomboids
    C. pectoralis
    D. erector spinae

M 580. In massaging the chest
    A. put pillows under the arms
    B. keep slight flexion at the knees
    C. client should be on back
    D. all of the above

M   **581.** During a massage of the abdomen, the patient should
         A. have hip flexors and abdominal muscles relaxed
         B. be on his or her side to relax
         C. be draped completely
         D. none of the above

M   **582.** In massaging the upper extremity,
         A. care should be taken at the joints
         B. popping of joints should be avoided
         C. stroke from distal to proximal along the bracioradialis
         D. all of the above

B/E   **583.** A massage therapist can get professional liability insurance from
         A. Prudential Insurance Company
         B. American Massage Therapy Association (AMTA)
         C. U.S. Health Care
         D. all of the above

M   **584.** In massaging the Achilles tendon,
         A. concentrate on cross-fiber friction
         B. one hand massages the foot, while the other hand flexes the foot
         C. avoid bimanual stroking
         D. lift leg up first

M   **585.** Massage to the popliteal area requires
         A. firm deep friction
         B. gentle working of the gastrocnemius tendon heads
         C. complete avoidance of space
         D. petrissage only

AP   **586.** Basal metabolic rate (BMR) is best determined
         A. after a heavy meal
         B. after a long period of exercise
         C. at rest, awake, and after a fast of approximately 12 hours
         D. while asleep and after a fast of at least 12 hours

AP   **587.** The invisible circulation of vital energy is called
   A. chi
   B. regulating channel
   C. Hseuh
   D. Yin and Yang

AP   **588.** The direction of energy flow of Yin is
   A. down from the head area to the foot
   B. down toward the chest
   C. across the chi
   D. up the chest to hand

M   **589.** The *Bindegewebsmassage* is a variation of massage technique that is based on
   A. massaging the connective tissue under the skin
   B. cross-fiber friction
   C. polarity
   D. none of the above

P   **590.** Dicke includes the disabilities that respond well to *Bindegewebsmassage* as
   A. epicondylitis
   B. scars
   C. lumbago
   D. all of the above

M   **591.** A massage stroke that ends with a "hook-on" is
   A. Traeger
   B. acupressure
   C. *Bindegewebsmassage*
   D. Swedish

AP   **592.** Which of the following play (plays) a role in wound healing and tissue repair?
   A. Age
   B. Blood circulation
   C. Nutrition and vitamins
   D. All of the above

M   **593.** In massage, it is important to
       A. break touch with the client
       B. apply oil over the entire body
       C. maintain contact with the client throughout
       D. prepare the client in a prone position

M   **594.** In massaging the body, it is important to
       A. drape all parts of the body
       B. expose only the part to be massaged
       C. cover the entire body with a sheet
       D. stand still while delivering technique

M   **595.** Friction can sometimes be classified as
       A. compression
       B. hacking
       C. cupping
       D. percussion

P   **596.** In difficult joint movement, the main objective is
       A. active assistive joint movement
       B. passive joint movements
       C. active resistive joint movement
       D. range of motion

P   **597.** Massage therapy is the best method of locating
       A. pain
       B. muscle dysfunction
       C. soft tissue dysfunction
       D. all of the above

M   **598.** Kneading includes all of the following **EXCEPT**
       A. rolling
       B. fulling
       C. petrissage
       D. friction

P   **599.** In runner's cramp, the massage treatment is
       A. ice application
       B. compression on stress points
       C. cross-fiber friction and shaking calf
       D. all of the above

P   **600.** Fibrosis in muscle may be the result of
      A. trauma or strain
      B. poor healing
      C. infection
      D. congestion in the tissues

Practice Test Questions 4

Answers and Discussion

451. **(D)** Iron is a mineral that is part of the hemoglobin in the RBC. *(Ref. 8, p. 848)*

452. **(B)** Any opening on the skin that doesn't heal could be cancer. *(Ref. 2, p. 258)*

453. **(A)** The blood can artificially be filtered of wastes by a method called hemodialysis. *(Ref. 8, p. 891)*

454. **(B)** The Amma bioenergy system is a series of complex channels throughout the body and organs. *(Ref. 12, p. 70)*

455. **(C)** Urine is processed in the cortex and medulla, collects in the pelvis passage to the ureter tube, which is connected to the bladder, and moves out the urethra. *(Ref. 8, p. 891)*

456. **(D)** Microscopically, the nephron is the functional unit that filters the blood. *(Ref. 8, p. 867)*

457. **(A)** Treatment with hot or cold application should not be given if a contraindication is present. *(Ref. 2, p. 471)*

458. **(D)** The heart, spleen, lung, kidney, and liver, as well as the seasons, the climate, and emotions are all associated with the five-pointed star of the elements. *(Ref. 12, p. 21)*

459. (B) The diffusion of water is called osmosis. A concentration gradient difference forces this function. *(Ref. 8, p. 905)*

460. (A) Swelling can be reduced by ice packs. *(Ref. 2, p. 467)*

461. (C) The somatic cells in humans contain 46 chromosomes or 23 pairs. Six cells contain 23 chromosomes. *(Ref. 8, p. 927)*

462. (C) One wellness component is taking care of the body through nutrition to help prevent fatigue and mood changes from cravings. *(Ref. 11, pp. 382–383)*

463. (B) After a thorough history intake and verbal interview, the therapist can develop a plan of action. *(Ref. 11, p. 15)*

464. (C) The pain-spasm-pain cycle is a result of restricted movement caused by trauma, strain, or injury to the bone, muscle, tendon, or joint. The muscle spasm contracts the muscle that becomes ischemic and that in turn stimulates the pain receptors in the muscle. *(Ref. 11, p. 94)*

465. (C) Friction of the cross-fibers is an excellent method to break down well-healed scar adhesions. *(Ref. 5, p. 83)*

466. (D) Vitamin D is essential for the absorption of calcium and phosphorous from the stomach. *(Ref. 8, p. 850)*

467. (C) Light massage to the knee area is beneficial, especially if there is edema. *(Ref. 5, p. 101)*

468. (B) The thyroid gland secretes the thyroid hormone, which aids in determining the basal metabolic rate (BMR). *(Ref. 8, p. 855)*

469. (C) The lung (L) meridian is the one with the most vital energy. *(Ref. 5, p. 135)*

470. (D) When the skeletal muscles contract, the body temperature rises. *(Ref. 8, p. 854)*

471. (D) The acronym HIV stands for human immunodeficiency virus. *(Ref. 8, p. 712)*

472. (B) The average volume of blood in an adult is 5 liters. *(Ref. 8, p. 630)*

473. (C) Different organs and parts of the body respond to reflex zones in the hands and feet. *(Ref. 5, p. 255)*

474. (C) The dense connective tissue includes tendons, ligaments, and elastic connective tissue. *(Ref. 8, p. 110)*

475. (A) Cartilage is a connective tissue that has few or no blood vessels or nerves. *(Ref. 8, p. 110)*

476. (C) The sphenoid bone is the keystone of the cranial floor because it articulates with many bones and is a common area for a headache massage. *(Ref. 8, p. 176)*

477. (A) Lordosis is a lumbar curvation of the spine due to poor posture, pregnancy, obesity, or rickets. *(Ref. 8, p. 195)*

478. (C) The cervical vertebra is part of the axial skeleton. *(Ref. 3, p. 22)*

479. (C) The glenoid cavity is where the scapula and humerus articulate. *(Ref. 8, p. 200)*

480. (D) Depending on your weight, the muscle is usually about 40–50% of the total. *(Ref. 8, p. 238)*

481. (A) Only light massage can benefit the ache and mucous secretion associated with the upper respiratory infections. *(Ref. 11, p. 407)*

482. (D) The chemoreceptor, proprioceptor, and baroreceptor are all involved in monitoring and controlling the rate of the heart. *(Ref. 8, p. 611)*

483. (C) External respiration is the gas exchange between the lungs and capillaries, and internal respiration is the gas exchange between the tissues. *(Ref. 8, p. 745)*

484. (D) The Heimlich maneuver (abdominal thrust) is the first-aid procedure to force air or water out of the trachea or lungs. *(Ref. 8, p. 761)*

485. (A) Asthma is the disorder that results in the narrowing of the airways as spasms of the smooth muscle close partially or completely (bronchoconstrictor). *(Ref. 8, p. 756)*

486. (B) The disbursement record comes from the checkbook, but columns separate each category of expenditure. *(Ref. 2, p. 633)*

487. (B) This is a record of credit extended to clients. *(Ref. 2, p. 637)*

488. (A) Accounts or businesses that extend you credit and bill you for amounts due. *(Ref. 2, p. 638)*

489. (C) Marketing is advertising, public relations, promotion, and client referrals. *(Ref. 2, p. 642)*

490. (B) Networking enhances the extension of the business. *(Ref. 2, p. 644)*

491. (D) A mission statement expresses the intent of the business and can be used for promotion. *(Ref. 2, p. 620)*

492. (C) Stockholders share in profits but are not legally responsible for the actions of the corporation. *(Ref. 2, p. 622)*

493. (B) Liability insurance is part of a homeowner's policy but may not cover business-related occurrences. *(Ref. 2, p. 626)*

494. (B) Good ethics provide guidelines for professional conduct, appearance, dignity, and legal requirements. *(Ref. 2, p. 628)*

495. (C) Massage techniques have an effect on reflex reaction to relieve pain. *(Ref. 2, p. 249)*

496. (B) Regular massage improves circulation, tones skin, softens lines, and prevents blemishes. *(Ref. 2, p. 252)*

497. (D) Shock is an absolute general contraindication to massage. *(Ref. 11, p. 393)*

498. (A) In about a four-hour period, a meal has been completely digested. *(Ref. 8, p. 844)*

499. (B) The movement of a joint from one articulation to the other. *(Ref. 2, p. 327)*

500. (B) Water in the form of ice, liquid, or steam vapor with massage has a therapeutic effect on the body. *(Ref. 2, p. 469)*

501. (B) Bubbles of carbon dioxide gas are produced by tablets. *(Ref. 2, p. 470)*

502. (A) Sponging is a procedure of hydrotherapy. *(Ref. 2, p. 471)*

503. (D) The skin and muscle and related areas have receptors that are stimulated from deep somatic pain. *(Ref. 11, p. 95)*

504. (C) Nerve sensitivity is reduced. *(Ref. 2, p. 472)*

505. (B) Blood vessels constrict initially after cold application. *(Ref. 2, p. 473)*

506. (C) The temperature for a hot bath is 100–115°F. *(Ref. 2, p. 473)*

507. (D) If three to five pounds of salt are added to a bath, the effect is that of bathing in sea water. *(Ref. 2, p. 473)*

508. (D) Since the pulse goes up in a hot bath, this may overwork the heart. *(Ref. 2, p. 474)*

509. (D) A steam room for cleansing and relaxing provides a Russian bath. *(Ref. 2, p. 481)*

510. (C) Extreme cold should be of short duration because the tissue temperature lowers. *(Ref. 2, p. 464)*

511. (C) Heat in a sauna room is always produced by a dry heat source of 120°F. *(Ref. 2, p. 463)*

512. (B) Water is able to cool or heat muscle tissue and change the body temperature. *(Ref. 2, p. 470)*

513. (B) Vomiting, diarrhea, and hypertension are all dehydrating mechanisms. *(Ref. 8, p. 907)*

514. **(D)** Spray showers have many hydrotherapeutic effects. *(Ref. 2, p. 462)*

515. **(C)** The tissue freezes if it is too cold too long. *(Ref. 2, p. 464)*

516. **(C)** Heat and cold are the most effective methods of promoting healing through circulation. *(Ref. 2, p. 469)*

517. **(C)** A sealable plastic bag makes an excellent ice pack. *(Ref. 2, p. 465)*

518. **(C)** These signs indicate sensitivity to skin to result in an allergic reaction. *(Ref. 2, p. 277)*

519. **(D)** A table should be comfortable with padding to absorb pressure applied by practitioners. *(Ref. 2, p. 274)*

520. **(D)** Many professionals and businesses hire massage therapists as employees. They include spas, hotels, doctors, and cruise ships. *(Ref. 11, p. 165)*

521. **(C)** To prevent fatigue, the palm of a hand should be flat on the table with arms straight. *(Ref. 2, p. 273)*

522. **(D)** In order to market a massage business effectively, the best places to advertise are the local newspaper, mail flyers, or the classified section of the phone book. *(Ref. 10, pp. 47–49)*

523. **(B)** A multiposition table is good for the elderly or disabled and when more than one person uses the table. *(Ref. 2, p. 274)*

524. **(B)** Mineral oils are not recommended because they are petroleum-based, dry the skin, and clog pores. *(Ref. 2, p. 276)*

525. **(A)** Mild oils, such as sesame and almond, are appropriate and easy to work with. *(Ref. 2, p. 276)*

526. **(B)** These are major nerves, blood vessels, and vital organs that are exposed to deep pressure and can cause possible injury. *(Ref. 2, p. 265)*

527. (A) Any visit outside an office—to a home or hospital—is an outcall. *(Ref. 2, p. 269)*

528. (A) The temperature of the room must be warm enough for the client and cool enough for the practitioner. *(Ref. 2, p. 272)*

529. (D) Soft natural light or indirect light is most desirable, especially for the eyes. *(Ref. 2, p. 272)*

530. (B) Injuries that cause inflammation to an area should not be massaged. *(Ref. 2, p. 4)*

531. (A) By working on areas that have been injured or affected by over-exercising, healing and circulation are improved. *(Ref. 2, pp. 507–508)*

532. (D) The mechanical effects of massage are directly related to the physical strokes and techniques used. *(Ref. 2, p. 506)*

533. (D) These strokes are generally used at the end and create a calming effect. *(Ref. 2, p. 312)*

534. (D) Everyone concerned should be aware that safety and personal hygiene are essential to a healthy atmosphere. *(Ref. 2, p. 287)*

535. (B) Good ethics and professional conduct are necessary. *(Ref. 2, p. 629)*

536. (D) Professional and ethical behavior does not include sexual activities under any circumstances. *(Ref. 2, p. 644)*

537. (D) Use of palpation can help to assess client condition before any massage is attempted. *(Ref. 11, p. 371)*

538. (A) It is important to be clear and honest with clients without giving unrealistic expectations. *(Ref. 2, p. 29)*

539. (A) Self-motivation means to make sacrifices when necessary. *(Ref. 2, p. 30)*

540. (C) Good planning and performance are assets for success. *(Ref. 2, p. 30)*

541. (D) Learning about new aspects of the field of massage as a health science is important. *(Ref. 2, p. 27)*

542. (A) Ethical conduct provides the client confidence in the place of business. *(Ref. 2, p. 26)*

543. (B) Business hours that accommodate clients are important for a professional image. *(Ref. 2, p. 30)*

544. (B) Individual ethics become part of the professional code of ethics. *(Ref. 2, p. 26)*

545. (B) Communicate in a confidential and professional manner without exposing personal matters. *(Ref. 2, p. 27)*

546. (A) Perform services for which you are qualified; for all others, refer clients to medical professionals. *(Ref. 2, p. 26)*

547. (A) A clean, neat, and attractive business is essential for a professional impression. *(Ref. 2, p. 27)*

548. (D) Potential disease or infection can be transmitted when administering first aid. *(Ref. 1, p. 29)*

549. (C) Ethics are standards of acceptable and professional behavior. *(Ref. 2, p. 629)*

550. (D) Call 911 or EMS. Talk to the person to get a response. *(Ref. 1, p. 29)*

551. (D) According to the IRS, self-employed individuals must make quarterly tax payments. *(Ref. 2, p. 627)*

552. (D) Check ABCs (airway, breathing, and circulation) and administer first aid. *(Ref. 1, p. 19)*

553. (B) Moist heat packs transfer heat to body parts by conduction. *(Ref. 2, p. 463)*

554. (C) The initial effect of cold is chilling the skin and contracting the blood vessels to limit swelling. *(Ref. 2, p. 472)*

555. **(B)** Local circulation is increased, chronic pain is relieved, and healing is aided. *(Ref. 2, p. 469)*

556. **(D)** Biofeedback, breathing for relaxation, and visualization are all stress reducers. *(Ref. 2, pp. 602–605)*

557. **(D)** Rescue breathing requires tilting the head, pinching the nose, and breathing into the mouth twice. *(Ref. 1, p. 199)*

558. **(C)** In CPR the pulse is checked at the carotid artery at side of neck. *(Ref. 1, p. 203)*

559. **(D)** For heat cramps, never give coffee, alcohol, or medication. Cool the person down at the neck, groin, and armpits. *(Ref. 1, p. 156)*

560. **(C)** A person who experiences heat stroke or cramps should be allowed to rest and get cool. *(Ref. 1, p. 158)*

561. **(B)** Protect the victim from injury during a seizure. *(Ref. 1, p. 169)*

562. **(C)** The first sign of a person choking is that he or she cannot answer. *(Ref. 1, p. 199)*

563. **(B)** To administer CPR correctly, place the hands on the end of sternum. *(Ref. 1, p. 204)*

564. **(A)** CPR can be administered to a victim who is not breathing or does not have a cardiac pulse. *(Ref. 1, p. 205)*

565. **(C)** Clutching the neck between the thumb and index finger is the universal distress signal of a choking victim. *(Ref. 13, p. 42)*

566. **(D)** The procedure for the Heimlich maneuver is to stand behind the victim and apply subdiaphragmatic thrusts into the abdomen with the fists. *(Ref. 13, p. 42)*

567. **(C)** Dizziness and numbness of the arm or leg usually on one side are the signs of a stroke. *(Ref. 13, p. 26)*

568. **(D)** In CPR it is important to pinch off the nostrils, tilt the head back, and observe the victim's chest. *(Ref. 13, p. 37)*

569. (C) Always turn an unconscious victim on the back before administering CPR, unless victim is vomiting. *(Ref. 13, p. 48)*

570. (D) Deep breathing exercise is a method to aid stress-related activities. *(Ref. 2, p. 602)*

571. (D) Yoga enhances muscle control, breathing, and relaxation and complements massage treatment. *(Ref. 2, p. 603)*

572. (D) Meditation is treatment for stimulating the flow of natural healing forces, as well as receiving subliminal messages. *(Ref. 5, p. 50)*

573. (C) Trigger point therapy palpates small areas of hypertonicity in the muscle associated with myofascial pain, and requires gentle stretching at the end. *(Ref. 11, p. 101)*

574. (D) Good massage techniques include checking patient comfort, even pressure when stroking, and good body positioning. *(Ref. 5, p. 71)*

575. (A) Knuckling and stroking are variations of effleurage. *(Ref. 5, p. 73)*

576. (D) The petrissage stroke varies as a V hand position, open and closed C position, and a one-handed petrissage. *(Ref. 5, p. 78)*

577. (D) The universal precautions were issued to prevent the spread of bacteria and virus. Therefore, contact with the client's blood, urine, feces and vomit should be avoided. *(Ref. 11, p. 113)*

578. (D) Cross-fiber manipulation is a variation of friction to mobilize the tissue under the skin. *(Ref. 5, p. 84)*

579. (C) The back does not contain the pectoralis muscle, which is the primary chest muscle. *(Ref. 5, p. 98)*

580. (D) For a chest massage, it is important to flex the knees and place a pillow under the arms, with the client supine. *(Ref. 5, p. 97)*

581. (A) Always relax the hip flexors and abdominal muscles when massaging the abdominal area. *(Ref. 5, p. 97)*

582. (D) When massaging the upper limbs, care should be taken with the movement of the joints and strokes should go from distal to proximal along the bracioradialis. *(Ref. 5, pp. 98–100)*

583. (B) Malpractice insurance is essential for a massage therapist. Professional organizations, such as AMTA, can provide liability protection. *(Ref. 11, p. 167)*

584. (B) For the Achilles tendon, massage the foot with one hand and flex the foot with the other hand. *(Ref. 5, p. 104)*

585. (B) The popliteal area of the posterior leg should be gently massaged due to the presence of blood vessels and nerves. *(Ref. 5, p. 102)*

586. (C) The best time to determine the basal metabolic rate is when a person is rested but awake, after a fast of 12 hours. *(Ref. 8, p. 853)*

587. (A) The chi is the Chinese word for the energy flow of the meridian. *(Ref. 5, p. 136)*

588. (D) The energy flow of Yin is on the upper body anterior side, up the chest to the hand. *(Ref. 5, p. 139)*

589. (A) The massage that concentrates on the connective tissue under the skin is the *Bindegewebsmassage. (Ref. 5, p. 220)*

590. (D) Many diseases and disorders respond well to the *Bindegewebsmassage,* such as epicondylitis, scars, and lumbago. *(Ref. 5, p. 222)*

591. (C) A characteristic stroke of the *Bindegewebsmassage* is the "hook-on." *(Ref. 5, p. 226)*

592. (D) The healing and repair of tissue depend on age, the amount of circulation, and vitamin and mineral levels. *(Ref. 8, pp. 122–123)*

593. (C) Strokes should be continuous and maintained without breaks in contact. The client can become startled with reestablishing contact. *(Ref. 2, p. 373)*

594. (B) Expose the area to be massaged, but keep the rest of body draped for privacy and professionalism. *(Ref. 2, p. 372)*

595. (A) Compression is a form of friction by rhythmical pumping directly into the muscle perpendicular to the body part. *(Ref. 2, p. 319)*

596. (A) In difficult ROM by the client, assistance may be provided by the therapist to move the body part. *(Ref. 2, p. 325)*

597. (D) Muscle soft tissue dysfunction and pain are symptoms that massage therapy treats. *(Ref. 2, p. 329)*

598. (D) Friction is a form of massage that moves superficial layers against deep layers, whereas kneading pulls and lifts flesh away from bone. *(Ref. 2, p. 315)*

599. (D) When the muscle goes into spasm and cramping results, ice, compression, and cross-fiber friction to contracted muscle provide considerable relief, as well as stretching the spasmed muscle. *(Ref. 2, p. 529)*

600. (A) Fibrosis is located in the muscle fascia and can be caused by strain, aging, or inflammation. *(Ref. 2, p. 557)*

Comprehensive Simulated Exam

1. The sequences and directions of Swedish massage strokes are most adapted to which anatomical or physiological situation?
   A. Muscle attachments
   B. Subcutaneous adipose tissue
   C. Autonomic nervous system
   D. Lymph drainage and venous return

2. Which **BEST** describes the effects of massage therapy?
   A. Increase venous and lymph flow
   B. Increase venous, decrease arterial flow
   C. Decrease venous and lymph flow
   D. Decrease venous, increase lymph flow

3. When massaging the thigh in the supine position, which muscle is involved?
   A. Hamstrings
   B. Quadriceps
   C. Gluteals
   D. Gastrocnemius

4. Massage is contraindicated for which of the following conditions?
  A. High blood pressure
  B. Constipation
  C. Keloid scar
  D. Adhesions

5. The iliopsoas flexes the hip because of its insertion on the
  A. femur
  B. greater trochanter
  C. lesser trochanter
  D. iliac crest

6. The tricuspid valve is found between the
  A. right atrium and right ventricle
  B. left ventricle and aorta
  C. left ventricle and right ventricle
  D. right atrium and left atrium

7. Which is a **TRUE** statement concerning Golgi tendon apparatus?
  A. Found in joint capsules
  B. Detects overall tension in tendon
  C. Originates in Purkinje fibers
  D. Activated by bagel reflex

8. Which muscles are adductors?
  A. Pectoralis and deltoid
  B. Pectoralis and latissimus dorsi
  C. Deltoid and latissimus dorsi
  D. Biceps and deltoids

9. Which muscle would be paralyzed if the sciatic nerve were severed?
  A. Trapezius
  B. Biceps femoris
  C. Gluteus maximus
  D. Erector spinae

10. Which most accurately describes the meridian system?
  A. Energy pathway moving randomly through the body
  B. Energy pathway moving superficially
  C. Energy pathway that doesn't affect organs
  D. 12 meridians and 2 vessels are pathways in which energy moves toward the surface of the body affecting organs

11. The best massage stroke to be used on a chronic sprain is
    A. transverse friction
    B. effleurage
    C. pick-up
    D. tapotement

12. Which condition is present when there is an injury of the ulna nerve at the elbow?
    A. Inability to flex fingers fully
    B. Spasticity
    C. Flaccidity
    D. Spasms

13. The only joint where the axial skeleton articulates with the appendicular skeleton is
    A. sternoclavicular
    B. glenohumeral
    C. sternoscapular
    D. scapularclavicular

14. What muscle is not part of the rotator cuff?
    A. Supraspinatus
    B. Infraspinatus
    C. Teres major
    D. Teres minor

15. Precision muscle testing, passive positioning, directional massage, and deep pressure are the physical techniques used in
    A. SMB
    B. TMJ
    C. NMF
    D. PBF

16. Acupuncture, *shiatsu,* polarity, and reflexology are examples of
    A. energetic manipulation
    B. behavioral barometer
    C. reactive circuits
    D. systematic massage

17. Lymph massage procedures begin at the
    A. tendons
    B. left thoracic lymph duct
    C. right thoracic lymph duct
    D. immune system

18. Cross-fiber massage must be applied in which direction to the fibers?
    A. Horizontally
    B. At right angles
    C. Triangularly
    D. Trapezoidally

19. Cold applied for therapeutic purposes is called
    A. cryptology
    B. cryotherapy
    C. ignorance
    D. cool ice

20. Thorough assessment of a client's condition reveals any
    A. lies
    B. weight gains
    C. credit gaps
    D. contraindications

21. Psychological benefits of massage include reduced tension and fatigue, calmer nerves, and
    A. therapeutics
    B. renewed energy
    C. improved circulation
    D. spasms

22. Friction, percussion, and vibration are techniques that
    A. stimulate
    B. relax
    C. strengthen
    D. weaken

23. The kneading technique in which the practitioner attempts to grasp tissue and gently lift and spread it out is called
    A. fulling
    B. pulling
    C. spreading
    D. nudging

24. Pressing one superficial layer of tissue against a deeper layer of tissue in order to flatten the deeper layer is called
    A. rolling
    B. spreading
    C. friction
    D. ironing

25. Nerve trunks and centers are sometimes chosen as sites for the application of
    A. rolling
    B. rocking
    C. pressure
    D. vibration

26. A bath with a temperature of 85°F to 95°F is considered
    A. cool
    B. cold
    C. tepid
    D. hot

27. The procedure that uses a bouncing movement to improve the flow of lymph through the entire system is called lymphatic
    A. bounce
    B. sway
    C. purging
    D. pump manipulation

28. The attempt to bring the structure of the body into alignment around a central axis is called
    A. structural integration
    B. trauma
    C. alignment
    D. adjustment

29. Realignment of muscular and connective tissue and reshaping the body's physical posture is called
  A. adjustment
  B. centering
  C. Rolfing
  D. posturing

30. A hyperirritable spot that is painful when compressed is called a (an)
  A. trigger point
  B. pain point
  C. ampule
  D. Rolfing

31. Relieving soreness, tension, and stiffness benefits which system?
  A. Muscular
  B. Skeletal
  C. Respiratory
  D. Excretory

32. In which directions do Yin meridians flow?
  A. Superior to inferior
  B. Inferior to superior
  C. Lateral to medial
  D. Medial to lateral

33. Injuries that have a gradual onset or reoccur often are called
  A. sprains
  B. occupational
  C. acute
  D. chronic

34. A sudden involuntary contraction of a muscle is called a (an)
  A. levator
  B. proximal
  C. isometric
  D. spasm

35. An exercise in which you imagine turning a large wheel is called
   A. the wheel
   B. grinding corn
   C. grounding
   D. centering

36. If a client's condition is outside the massage technician's scope of practice, the technician should
   A. schedule extra sessions
   B. refer the client to the proper professional
   C. take more training
   D. read textbooks

37. Describing how the organs or body parts function and relate to one another is the study of
   A. physiology
   B. histology
   C. anatomy
   D. pathology

38. The branch of biology concerned with the microscopic structure of living tissues is
   A. physiology
   B. histology
   C. anatomy
   D. pathology

39. Which meridians are innervated by massaging the medial thigh?
   A. KI, LIV, SP
   B. GB, ST, SP
   C. LIV, ST, KI
   D. GB, LIV, KI

40. A relaxing atmosphere for massage may be created with
   A. clothing
   B. music
   C. wall coverings
   D. carpet

41. Cardiac muscle tissue occurs only in the
  A. liver
  B. stomach
  C. heart
  D. mouth

42. Blood is an example of
  A. cardiac tissue
  B. connective tissue
  C. nerve tissue
  D. striated muscles

43. In anatomy, the sagittal plane divides the body into left and right parts by an imaginary line running
  A. vertically
  B. horizontally
  C. diagonally
  D. circularly

44. Cancer is a disease that can be spread through the
  A. genes
  B. lymphatic and blood system
  C. endocrine system
  D. digestive system

45. The general effects of percussion movements are to tone the muscles by
  A. vibration
  B. friction
  C. kneading
  D. hacking, cupping, slapping, beating

46. The Traeger method uses movement exercises called
  A. gymnastics
  B. mentastics
  C. spirals
  D. athletics

47. Aligning major body segments through manipulation of connective tissue is the
   A. Rolfing method
   B. Traeger method
   C. Palmer method
   D. reflexology method

48. The idea that the stimulation of particular body points affects other areas is called
   A. chiropractic
   B. reflexology
   C. Rolfing
   D. touching

49. Applied kinesiology methods are designed to relieve stress on muscles and
   A. joints
   B. bones
   C. ligaments
   D. internal organs

50. To reduce adhesions and fibrosis, which movement is used?
   A. Cross-fiber friction
   B. Wringing
   C. Pressing
   D. Squeezing

51. Massage is not performed on an area that is
   A. bleeding
   B. swollen
   C. burned
   D. all of the above

52. The Tendino-Muscle Channels of the lung pass through muscles of the chest and arm that include
   A. pectorals
   B. biceps brochii
   C. diaphragm
   D. all of the above

53. Severe strain of the trapezius and deltoid muscles is called
   A. racquetball shoulder
   B. tennis elbow
   C. skier's snap
   D. bowler's break

54. Overstretching of the gracilis and adductor muscle on the inner thigh results from
   A. soccer
   B. tennis
   C. horseback riding
   D. bowling

55. Severe varicose veins is a (an) _____ for massage.
   A. Indication
   B. Circulation
   C. Embolus
   D. Contraindication

56. A survivor of abuse can benefit from massage by
   A. feeling a sense of safeness
   B. releasing or letting go some of the abuse
   C. retrieving memory
   D. all of the above

57. Which meridian is lateral to the midsagittal line of the posterior cervical vertebrae?
   A. Governing vessel
   B. Triple warmer
   C. Stomach
   D. Bladder

58. What forms the outer layer of the anterior and lateral abdominal wall?
   A. Rectus abdominis
   B. Transversalis
   C. Serratus anterior
   D. External oblique

59. The primary flexor of the distal phalange of the fingers is
  A. flexor carpi ulnaris
  B. pollices longus
  C. flexor digitorum profundus
  D. flexor carpi radialis

60. A basic pattern of energy for the stomach channel is
  A. 7 a.m. to 9 a.m.
  B. 7 p.m. to 9 p.m.
  C. 3 a.m. to 5 a.m.
  D. 3 p.m. to 5 p.m.

61. Sciatic nerve damage diminishes ability to
  A. flex the hip
  B. flex the knee
  C. adduct the hip
  D. adbuct the hip

62. Deep strokes and kneading techniques can cause an increase in
  A. vasoconstriction
  B. blood flow
  C. diastolic arterial pressure
  D. systolic arterial pressure

63. What **BEST** describes the technique of Rolfing?
  A. Reflex zone therapy
  B. German massage
  C. Structural integration
  D. Connective tissue massage

64. Manipulation of the occipital regions of the neck primarily affects
  A. HT and BL meridians
  B. CO and KI meridians
  C. BL and GB meridians
  D. ST and SP meridians

65. Facial paralysis is due to a lesion in which cranial nerve?
  A. III
  B. VI
  C. VII
  D. VIII

66. Which muscle elevates and depresses the scapula?
   A. Trapezius
   B. Latissimus dorsi
   C. Rhomboids
   D. All of the above

67. With the elbow flexed, which muscle supinates the palm?
   A. Pronator
   B. Supinator
   C. Quadrator
   D. Brachialis

68. Deep friction massage works **BEST** if it is applied
   A. directly over problem area
   B. proximal to problem area
   C. distal to problem area
   D. around the problem area

69. The cupping technique is **BEST** suited for
   A. acute bronchitis
   B. cancer of the lungs
   C. bronchiectasis
   D. acute tracheitis

70. The last step in clot formation is
   A. prothrombin to thrombin
   B. fibrinogen to fibrin
   C. platelet formation
   D. tissue trauma

71. The exchange of O_2 and CO_2 takes place in the
   A. alveoli
   B. bronchi
   C. bronchioles
   D. pleural cavity

72. The temperature range for hot immersion baths is **BEST** at
   A. 85°F–95°F
   B. 100°F–110°F
   C. 125°F–150°F
   D. 130°F–140°F

73. To treat the seventh cranial palsy (Bell's palsy), brisk friction kneading should be done
   A. from the mandible to hairline vertically
   B. from the hairline to mandible
   C. transversely with both hands
   D. not at all

74. The therapeutic benefit of friction is
   A. local hyperemia
   B. lymphatic drainage
   C. tonification
   D. none of the above

75. In which directions do Yin meridians flow?
   A. Superior to inferior
   B. Inferior to superior
   C. Lateral to medial
   D. Medial to lateral

76. The best massage to use on a chronic sprain is
   A. effleurage
   B. pick-up
   C. transverse friction
   D. vibration

77. Which is a band of strong, fibrous tissue that connects the articular ends of bones and binds them together?
   A. Membrane
   B. Fascia
   C. Cancellous tissue
   D. Ligament

78. Which stroke most often begins and ends a massage?
   A. Effleurage
   B. Petrissage
   C. Friction
   D. Vibration

79. What is the first primary consideration before beginning massage treatment?
   A. Make sure the client is comfortable
   B. Make sure no jewelry is being worn
   C. Wash hands thoroughly
   D. Determine if contraindications are present

80. How should you vary massage treatment with the age of the patient?
   A. Progressively with increased age
   B. Shorter with increased age
   C. Shorter for very old and very young
   D. The same for any age

81. How should pressure be administered during effleurage?
   A. Even
   B. Heavy decreasing to light
   C. Intermittent
   D. Light to heavy

82. In oriental theory, Yin energy flows
   A. anterior to posterior
   B. dorsal to ventral
   C. inferior to superior
   D. superior to inferior

83. Massage can relieve pain without the use of
   A. imagery
   B. stimulation
   C. drugs, alcohol, or narcotics
   D. endorphins

84. Yoga is a form of meditation for
   A. good appetite
   B. muscle balance and relaxation
   C. dancing
   D. religion

85. In which massage technique should the fingers move tissue under the skin but not the skin itself?
   A. Tapotement
   B. Effleurage
   C. Vibration
   D. Friction

86. For which type of tissue is vibration the most unsuitable?
   A. Major nerve course
   B. Muscle origins
   C. Bony prominences
   D. Skeletal muscle

87. Hot compresses used immediately after injury do **NOT**
   A. increase blood flow
   B. reduce muscle spasm
   C. reduce swelling
   D. relieve pain

88. Which is the first step in beginning massage treatment?
   A. Apply lubricant
   B. Effleurage
   C. Determine contraindications
   D. Diagnose the patient

89. When giving CPR to a 6-year-old child, you use the
   A. heel of one hand
   B. heel of two hands
   C. fingers of one hand
   D. fingers of two hands

90. The popliteus muscle of the leg
   A. adducts
   B. extends
   C. plantar flexes the ankle
   D. medially rotates the tibia

91. First aid for acute soft tissue injuries involves RICE, which means
   A. ice
   B. rest and elevation
   C. compression
   D. all of the above

92. Massage treatment of the chest should **NEVER** be done over the
    A. ribs
    B. heart
    C. female nipples
    D. all of the above

93. Which aims most specifically to passively stretch muscle?
    A. Effleurage
    B. Friction
    C. Petrissage
    D. Tapotement

94. Massage benefits lymph flow **BEST** when strokes are
    A. away from the heart
    B. toward the heart
    C. heavy in both directions
    D. in certain local areas

95. Shinsplint syndrome affects the
    A. lateral malleplus
    B. periosterum around the tibia
    C. fibula
    D. all of the above

96. The thoracic duct drains the
    A. entire body below the ribs
    B. head, neck, chest, left limbs
    C. largest lymph drainage of the body
    D. all are true

97. Which muscle is innervated by the axillary nerve?
    A. Deltoid
    B. Brachial
    C. Pectoralis major
    D. None of the above

98. Which is best to prevent adhesions in muscle tissue?
    A. Friction and effleurage
    B. Friction and petrissage
    C. Friction and tapotement
    D. Friction only

99. Petrissage beginning just distal to the medial condyle and moving proximal to the gluteal fold affects what muscles?
  A. Anterior adductors
  B. Medial hamstrings
  C. Quadriceps
  D. Deltoids

100. In tapping a large area of the body, which massage maneuver is used?
  A. Percussion
  B. Friction
  C. Effleurage
  D. Petrissage

101. Which condition is always a contraindication for massage?
  A. Muscle spasm
  B. Phlebitis
  C. Rheumatoid arthritis
  D. Edema

102. The main purpose of deep transverse friction is to
  A. separate muscle fibers
  B. lengthen muscle
  C. shorten muscle fibers
  D. minimize pain

103. Adult body temperature is higher than normal at
  A. 37°C
  B. 98°F
  C. 98.6°F
  D. 39°C

104. The triple warmer controls
  A. assimilation, digestion, elimination
  B. assimilation, digestion, skin temperature regulation
  C. digestion, elimination, skin temperature regulation
  D. elimination, digestion, nervous system

105. What plantarflexes and everts the foot?
    A. Tibialis anterior
    B. Gastrocnemius
    C. Plantaris
    D. Peroneus longus

106. Which muscle inserts into the iliotibial band?
    A. Gluteus maximus
    B. Quadratus femoris
    C. Gluteus medias
    D. Tensor fascia latae

107. Contraindications for hydrotherapy include all of the following **EXCEPT**
    A. kidney infection
    B. cold
    C. high or low blood pressure
    D. skin infection

108. Massage therapy is used in pain management for
    A. cardiac and terminal cancer patients
    B. posttrauma patients
    C. postsurgical patients
    D. all of the above

109. Connective tissue massage (CTM) is a useful technique for
    A. preparing for surgery
    B. psychoemotional status
    C. loosening tissue following surgery or trauma
    D. controlling pain

110. The primary physiological effect of massage therapy includes all of the following **EXCEPT**
    A. delivery of oxygen to cells
    B. clearance of metabolic waste and by-product of tissue damage
    C. increase in blood and lymph circulation
    D. increase in interstitial fluid and hydrostatic pressure

111. Vodder's manual lymph drainage (MLD) was developed for the specific purpose of
   A. promoting lymph flow from tissue
   B. eliminating the pneumatic cuff
   C. decreasing urine output
   D. increasing erythrocyte count

112. Fibrosis, the formation of abnormal collagenous connective tissue, is best treated by
   A. deep friction massage
   B. passive movements
   C. kneading
   D. all of the above

113. The analgesic effect of ice massage is to
   A. block pain-impulse conduction
   B. reroute pain
   C. decrease ROM
   D. eliminate pain

114. Business expenses can include
   A. business cards and advertising
   B. professional clothes and linens
   C. license, insurance, and memberships
   D. all of the above

115. Client files are important because
   A. the Internal Revenue Service requires record keeping
   B. practitioner's must keep well informed of client's needs
   C. you have documented your "work" on clients
   D. all of the above

116. Good bookkeeping for healing arts professionals can
   A. eliminate tracking sheets
   B. decrease bank statements
   C. increase petty cash funds
   D. increase legitimate tax deductions

117. If you are a self-employed massage therapist, you must file
   A. no returns
   B. only Schedule C—Profit or Loss form

    C. Form 1040 and Social Security Self-Employment Tax form
    D. B and C

118. Beneficial techniques to market professional skills include
    A. publications and presentations
    B. business cards and brochures
    C. donation of services
    D. all of the above

119. Good client records should include
    A. intake form
    B. intake, health information, treatment, and session notes
    C. client history
    D. payments received

120. A typical client intake form should include
    A. name and address
    B. name, address, occupation, physician, emergency number
    C. name, phone, hobbies
    D. name, marital status, children

121. Massage can be effective in all of the following **EXCEPT**
    A. facilitating rehabilitation
    B. inhibiting a psychological effect
    C. preparing healthy muscles for strenuous activity
    D. enhancing the healing process

122. The purpose of a lubricant when massaging is to
    A. keep the body greasy
    B. prevent blisters from forming
    C. cleanse the body for relaxation
    D. avoid uncomfortable friction between the therapist's hand and the patient's skin

123. The reflex effects of massage are the stimulation of
    A. motor neurons
    B. sensory receptors of skin and subcutaneous tissues
    C. synovial fluid at each joint
    D. chemotransmitter

124. The benefits of massage to the skin, with the aim of returning it to normal function, include
   A. slowing metabolism
   B. removal of excretory products and dead skin
   C. decrease of hair growth
   D. preventing scar tissue from forming

125. Endorphins, which act like morphine for pain relief, are released from the
   A. ANS
   B. midbrain
   C. limbic system and brain stem
   D. CNS

126. The purpose of effleurage in massage is
   A. relaxation
   B. ROM
   C. to search for spasms and spread lubricant
   D. to apply pressure to the spine

127. The kneading motion of petrissage serves to "milk" the muscle and
   A. remove waste products
   B. assist abnormal inactivity
   C. assist venous return
   D. all of the above

128. The Chinese consider the lung as the delicate organ because
   A. it is a delicate tissue
   B. it is the first organ to be injured by negative substances
   C. it cannot work without the heart
   D. all of the above

129. Which terms means "on the opposite side of the body"?
   A. Contralateral
   B. Distal
   C. Intermediate
   D. Proximal

130. Which element is needed for clotting and muscle contraction, and contributes to the hardness of teeth and bone?
  A. Calcium
  B. Hydrogen
  C. Iron
  D. Nitrogen

131. Jin Shin Do is an oriental therapy that is
  A. preventative rather than symptomatic in nature
  B. to strengthen our absorption of life energy
  C. acupressure with breathing and meditation
  D. all of the above

132. An energy balancing therapy that attempts to remove blockages and bring healing energy to the problem areas is called
  A. reflexology
  B. therapeutic touch
  C. Amma therapy
  D. myofascial release

133. A second-degree burn is characterized by
  A. involvement of the entire epidermis and possibly some of the dermis
  B. no loss of skin functions
  C. damage to most hair follicles and sweat glands
  D. never scarring

134. Which of the following is defined as the degeneration of cartilage that allows the bony ends to touch and that is usually associated with the elderly?
  A. Osteoarthritis
  B. Osteogenic sarcoma
  C. Osteomyelitis
  D. Osteopenia

135. The Amma therapy is a full-body manipulation of the Coetaneous Regions, twelve organ channels, governing and conception vessels as well as
  A. Tendino-Muscle Channels
  B. TS points
  C. Yin-Yang
  D. Qi of the Heaven

136. Which of the following joint classifications is described as freely movable?
   A. Amphiarthrosis
   B. Cartilaginous
   C. Diarthrosis
   D. Fibrous

137. Which facial muscle inserts into the mandible, angles of the mouth, and skin of the lower face?
   A. Buccinator
   B. Depressor labii inferior
   C. Levator labii superioris
   D. Platysma

138. What is the spinal nerve contribution that composes the brachial plexus?
   A. C_1–C_4; T_1
   B. C_5–C_8; T_1
   C. C_7–C_8; T_1
   D. T_2–T_{12}; L_1

139. The sciatic nerve is actually two nerves. Which nerves comprise the sciatic nerve?
   A. Common peroneal and pudendal
   B. Tibial and medial plantars
   C. Medial and lateral plantars
   D. Common peroneal and tibial

140. Which of the following is the major muscle involved in crossing one's leg?
   A. Gastrocnemius
   B. Rectus femoris
   C. Sartorius
   D. Semimembranosus

141. The cerebellum
   A. functions to maintain proper posture and equilibrium
   B. receives input from the motor cortex and basal ganglia
   C. receives input from proprioceptors in joints and muscles
   D. has all of the above characteristics

142. A critical principle of holistic health is that the mind and body
    A. are separate from the organs
    B. function independently
    C. is seen as a single entity
    D. forces the healing process

143. The blood type that is termed the "universal donor" is
    A. O
    B. A
    C. B
    D. AB

144. The most numerous formed element in the blood is the
    A. thrombocyte
    B. leukocyte
    C. erythrocyte
    D. monocyte

145. Which of the following is characteristic of the sympathetic nervous system?
    A. Decreased heart rate
    B. Constricted pupils
    C. Splitting of glycogen to glucose in the liver
    D. Constriction of the bronchioles

146. The Ki flow through the meridians is the
    A. Hara breathing meditation
    B. blockage
    C. universal life energy
    D. spirit

147. Which point(s) should be checked while practicing?
    A. Is the stance of good body positioning and height?
    B. Is the patient comfortable and relaxed?
    C. Is the pressure even throughout each stroke?
    D. All of the above

148. Variations of effleurage include
   A. knuckling and stroking
   B. backstroke and friction
   C. pressure and brushing
   D. wide angling and stroking

149. Variations of petrissage include
   A. one-handed petrissage
   B. open and closed C position
   C. V hand position
   D. all of the above

150. Adhesions of a well-healed scar can be broken down between skin tissue by applying
   A. vibration
   B. petrissage
   C. friction
   D. effleurage

Comprehensive Simulated Exam

Answer Key

1. D	**26.** C	**51.** D	**76.** C
2. A	**27.** D	**52.** D	**77.** D
3. B	**28.** A	**53.** A	**78.** A
4. A	**29.** C	**54.** C	**79.** D
5. C	**30.** A	**55.** D	**80.** C
6. A	**31.** A	**56.** D	**81.** D
7. B	**32.** B	**57.** D	**82.** C
8. B	**33.** D	**58.** D	**83.** C
9. B	**34.** D	**59.** C	**84.** B
10. D	**35.** A	**60.** A	**85.** D
11. A	**36.** B	**61.** B	**86.** C
12. C	**37.** A	**62.** B	**87.** C
13. A	**38.** B	**63.** C	**88.** C
14. C	**39.** A	**64.** C	**89.** A
15. A	**40.** B	**65.** C	**90.** D
16. A	**41.** C	**66.** A	**91.** D
17. C	**42.** C	**67.** B	**92.** C
18. B	**43.** A	**68.** D	**93.** A
19. B	**44.** B	**69.** C	**94.** B
20. D	**45.** D	**70.** B	**95.** B
21. B	**46.** B	**71.** A	**96.** B
22. A	**47.** A	**72.** B	**97.** A
23. A	**48.** B	**73.** A	**98.** A
24. C	**49.** D	**74.** A	**99.** B
25. D	**50.** A	**75.** B	**100.** A

101. B	**114.** D	**127.** C	**140.** C
102. A	**115.** D	**128.** B	**141.** D
103. D	**116.** D	**129.** A	**142.** C
104. C	**117.** C	**130.** A	**143.** A
105. D	**118.** D	**131.** D	**144.** C
106. D	**119.** B	**132.** C	**145.** C
107. B	**120.** B	**133.** A	**146.** C
108. D	**121.** B	**134.** A	**147.** D
109. C	**122.** D	**135.** A	**148.** A
110. D	**123.** B	**136.** C	**149.** D
111. A	**124.** B	**137.** D	**150.** C
112. D	**125.** C	**138.** B	
113. A	**126.** A	**139.** D	

References

The following references or books have been used by the National Certification Board for Therapeutic Massage and Bodywork (NCTMB) for development of the Certifying Examination, and have been used in preparation for review book content areas.

1. American Red Cross. *Standard First Aid.* St. Louis, MO: Mosby Lifeline, 1993.

2. Beck M. *The Theory and Practice of Therapeutic Massage.* Albany, NY: Milady Publishing Corporation, 1994.

3. Kapit W. and Laurence E. *The Anatomy Coloring Book.* New York, NY: HarperCollins, 1977.

4. Sohnen-Moe C. *Business Master,* 2nd ed. Tucson, AZ: Sohnen-Moe Associates, 1991.

5. Tappan FM. *Healing Massage Technique: Holistic, Classic, and Emerging Methods.* Norwalk, CT: Appleton & Lange, 1988.

6. Thomas CL (ed). *Taber's Cyclopedic Medical Dictionary,* 16th ed. Philadelphia, PA: FA Davis Co., 1989.

7. Thompson CW. *Manual of Structural Kinesiology,* 11th ed. St. Louis, MO: Times Mirror/Mosby College Publisher, 1988.

8. Tortora GJ and Grabowski SR. *Principles of Anatomy and Physiology,* 7th ed. New York: Harper & Row, 1993.

9. Yates J. *A Physician's Guide to Therapeutic Massage.* Vancouver, BC: Massage Therapists' Association of British Columbia, 1990.

The following references have been added to expand the exam question resources to add non-Western techniques and holistic and touch therapy modalities and to increase business, ethics, and clinical pathology questions.

10. Ashley. *Massage: A Career at Your Fingertips.* Brewster, NY: Enterprising Publishers, 1998.

11. Fritz. *Fundamentals of Therapeutic Massage.* St. Louis: Mosby Lifeline, 1995.

12. Sohn T. and R. *Amma Therapy: A Complete Textbook of Oriental Bodywork and Medical Priniciples.* Rochester, VT: Healing Arts Press, 1996.

13. Teaguarden. *Acupressure: Way of Health.* Jin Shin Do Japan Publishers, 1995.

14. Thompson. *Hands Heal: Documentation for Massage Therapy.* Self-published, 1993.

2. Hard Disk Installation from File Manager in Windows® 3. or 3.11

    a. Once the computer is started, insert the the MICROSTUDY disk marked INSTALL into the appropriate floppy drive.

    b. From File Manager, click on the floppy drive symbol where the MICROSTUDY INSTALL disk was inserted. Find the program file INSTALL.EXE and double click on it to start the installation.

    c. INSTALL copies of all required files from the designated floppy drive to the designated hard drive and its sub-directories, then create a MICROSTUDY icon within a MICROSTUDY program group.

    d. Start MICROSTUDY by double clicking with a mouse on the MICROSTUDY program icon in the MICROSTUDY group.

3. Hard Disk Installation from Start in Windows® 95

    a. Once the computer is started, insert the MICROSTUDY disk marked INSTALL into the appropriate floppy drive.

    b. Select Run from the Start Menu. Type A:\INSTALL or B:\INSTALL in the Command Line of Run, then press OK.

    c. INSTALL copies of all required files from the designated floppy drive to the designated hard drive and its sub-directories, then create a MICROSTUDY icon within a MICROSTUDY program group.

    d. Start MICROSTUDY by double clicking with a mouse on the MICROSTUDY program icon in the MICROSTUDY group.

4. Hard Disk Installation from Explorer in Windows® 95

    a. Once the computer is started, insert the MICROSTUDY disk marked INSTALL into the appropriate floppy drive.

    b. From Explorer, click on the floppy drive symbol in which the MICROSTUDY INSTALL disk was inserted. Find the program file INSTALL.EXE and double click on it to start installation.

    c. INSTALL copies of all required files from the designated floppy drive to the designated hard drive and its sub-directories, then create a MICROSTUDY icon within a MICROSTUDY group.

    d. Start MICROSTUDY by double clicking with a mouse on the MICROSTUDY program icon in the MICROSTUDY group.

ECTIONS FOR INSTALLING
MICROSTUDY®

MICROSTUDY® V3.2 FOR WINDOWS FEATURES

1. Quizzes consisting of chapter questions may be taken in the authors' original order or in a randomly scrambled order.

2. Follow-up tests are composed of missed questions.

3. Electronic notebook enables students' comments to be entered and saved while studying, then recalled later for review, modifying, or printing.

4. Customized comprehensive exams may be automatically built. These exams may be presented under NAPLEX simulation or in the standard MICROSTUDY simulated exam format.

5. Performance is monitored and a report card is assembled after each work session. Comprehensive exam statistics are tabulated and displayed for exam performance comparisons.

6. Digital timer shows elapsed study time.

7. Audio feedback that signals responses may be used.

8. A four-function memory calculator is available while studying.

MICROSTUDY® V3.2 FOR WINDOWS®
INSTALLATION AND STARTUP

1. Hard Disk Installation from Run in Windows® 3.1 or 3.11

   a. Once the computer is started, insert the MICROSTUDY disk marked INSTALL into the appropriate floppy drive.

   b. Select Run from under the File Menu. Type A:\INSTALL or B:\INSTALL in the Command Line of Run, then press OK.

   c. INSTALL copies of all required files from the designated floppy drive to the designated hard drive and its subdirectories, then create a MICROSTUDY icon within a MICROSTUDY program group.

   d. Start MICROSTUDY by double clicking with a mouse on the MICROSTUDY program icon in the MICROSTUDY group.